26 Ideas For Positive Change

By Debbie J Hagedorn

ISBN 978-0-9973480-3-3

Published by 721 Publishing
Cover Design Jeanine Henning

Dedication

On this day, February 19, 2017, I dedicate this book to my whys, Caroline and Theodore. May you always remember that anything is possible if you are willing to keep learning and make changes when needed. I love you, always and forever!

~ Mom

Disclaimer

The information provided in this book is designed to provide helpful information on the subjects discussed. This book is not meant to be used, nor should it be used, to diagnose or treat any medical condition. For diagnosis or treatment of any medical problem, consult your own physician. The publisher and author are not responsible for any specific health or allergy needs that may require medical supervision and are not liable for any damages or negative consequences from any treatment, action, application or preparation, to any person reading or following the information in this book. References are provided for informational purposes only and do not constitute endorsement of any websites or other sources. Readers should be aware that the websites listed in this book may change.

Table Of Contents

Introduction

Your life! It's busy. It's still about you, though, no matter how many nights you run for your kids. You deserve nothing less than the best. If you wish to make healthier choices in your life, but you simply cannot find time to research healthier options, or you've done some looking and find yourself overwhelmed with all of the options, fear not. I've listed out 26 areas in this book in an A to Z format, each of which offers simple ideas for positive change. You'll see them listed out in the table of contents. Choose the one that works for you this week. Choose another when you're ready again. Even though you're big, baby steps are okay. As long as you keep moving forward, all will be well! I'll be cheering you along each step of the way. You CAN do this! I believe in you.

How to Use This Book

26 Ideas For Positive Change offers 26 individual selections for you to choose from when starting on your journey to making healthier choices in your life. These selections are in an A to Z format and, while many are related to food choices, there are also those meant to quiet your mind and nurture your soul. There is no need to start at the beginning.

Instead, after looking through the Table of Contents, select the topic that resonates with YOU the most. In other words, which topic jumps out at you? Which topic is figuratively waving its hands and calling your name? Choose that one!

Your task at the end of each chapter is to journal. Write down any ideas about the topic that came to you while you were reading. If you decide to implement the topic, write down your target date to start. Setting your goals on paper is an important step and will help you achieve them! Add any other thoughts that seem important, too. Dismiss nothing. These ideas and thoughts are your intuition talking to you. It's time to listen carefully.

Read additional selections as time permits, all the while knowing these selections are offered by a mom who found it to be her passion to learn all she could about making healthier choices for her family. Every selection has made a positive difference in their lives. She hopes they will make a positive difference in yours, too!

Chapter 1 - Alternatives to Food Additives

If the majority of the food you buy is pre-packaged and not organic, the likelihood is that these foods contain chemical additives of one kind or another. Chemical additives include colors, artificial sweeteners, and preservatives. In theory, the colors make a food product more appealing to the consumer, the artificial sweeteners offer sweet flavor without the calories of traditional sugar, and preservatives do simply what their name suggests - preserve the food product so it doesn't spoil in your refrigerator, on your counter, or in your pantry.

On the surface, these seem like good ideas. The trouble is, these products are being linked more and more often to various behavioral and health ailments within the human body. Nearly every jar of pickles, many candies, and citrus sodas contains Yellow No. 5, known to cause allergic reactions including asthma and suspected as a trigger for hyperactivity and cancer.[1]

Aspartame, also known as NutraSweet, is currently being marketed as AminoSweet. An artificial sweetener by any other name is still a toxin and something you may wish to eliminate from your diet. This one in particular may cause headaches, hallucinations, and joint pain, to name a few potential side effects. Many years ago, it was listed by the Pentagon as a biochemical warfare agent.[2] Today, you will find it on the ingredients list of nearly every pack of chewing gum, diet soda, and a long list of other sugar-free products throughout the grocery store. It may even be hiding in vitamins and some prescription drugs your family is taking. Preservatives are often noted as such on the label. Common preservatives include sodium nitrate, found in cured and smoked meats, BHA, BHT, sulfites, and sulfur dioxide. Large amounts of cured meats in your diet may increase your risk of various cancers.[3] BHA & BHT have been related to behavioral changes and may cause cancer. Sulfites are allergenic and can be dangerous for someone with asthma. Sulfur dioxide is commonly found in dried fruits and juices. Currently prohibited on raw fruits and vegetables in the United States, sulfur dioxide is considered toxic and is also very dangerous to those with impaired lung function, whether from asthma, bronchitis, emphysema, or other conditions.[4]

So, what are the alternatives to these chemical additives? I will be the first to tell you the challenge is real. Mainstream grocery items will need to go by the wayside. Begin to replace your usual products with those having organic labels. You may find these in a "natural" food section or dispersed in and amongst the more familiar products. Choose whole foods from the outer perimeter of the store. Acceptable colorants come from beets, carrots, turmeric, and other actual foods. Stevia is an herb with amazing sweetening capabilities. Admittedly, it does have a taste different from cane sugar. In my opinion, though, the taste is acceptable, unlike the taste, and ongoing aftertaste, of aspartame.

If you weren't looking for a sugar replacement in the first place, then consider using products with cane sugar. You'll want to watch for "cane" in the ingredients, though, because there is danger in the simple "sugar" option, too. If it's not cane, the source

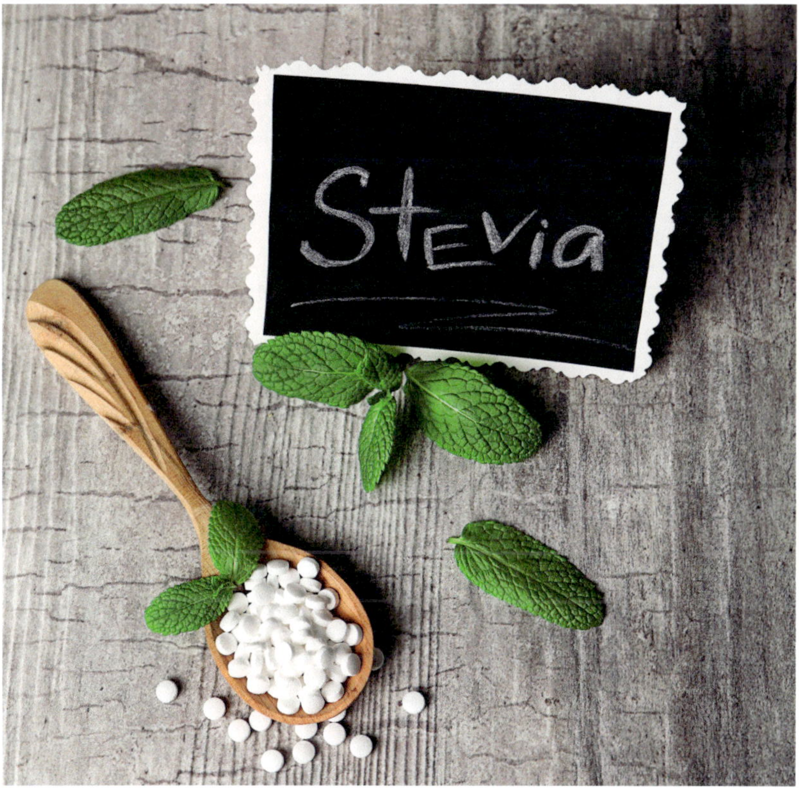

of sugar is likely sugar beets, and here in the United States, most of those beets have been genetically modified. That is a topic I'll discuss more thoroughly in Chapter 26 of this book.

Chapter 2 - Breathe Distress Away

There are many moments in a day. If you're at all like me, you would prefer to spend most of those in a positive, productive, easy-going state of mind. In thinking good thoughts, you'll find more good thoughts and things are on their way to you. The universal law of attraction insists this is true! The trouble is, not every moment is as calm and collected as you (or I!) may have hoped. In these off moments, don't despair - sanity is mere breaths away!
Emotional discomfort is simply an awareness that you are not in alignment with your true self. When you are feeling distress, mindful breathing WILL help relieve these negative feelings and bring your focus to the present moment. Mindful breathing will take the edge off of a dangerous situation and allow you to process information clearly. Mindful breathing will help you overcome nonstop feelings of worry and/or panic and give you moments of peace during which you are able to regain your sense of knowing that all will be well!
The process itself is simple. Stop in the midst of what is happening around you. You may choose to stay right where you are or find a quiet, safe space. Either will work, unless you're driving a moving vehicle! Close your eyes. Take a deep breath in through your nose. Once your lungs are full, hold this breath for two or three seconds. Release this breath through your mouth, pursing your lips as though you were drinking through a straw.

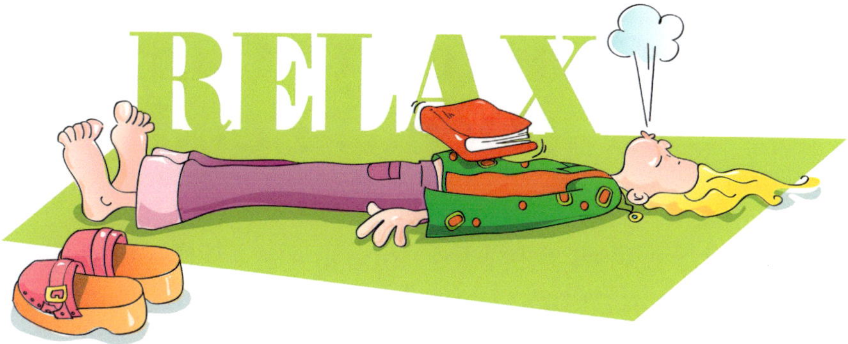

One key component to taking these breaths is to place your focus on the air that is moving into and out of your nose and your mouth. As far as how many breaths to take - continue breathing in this manner for 30 seconds. It is okay to do more or less, depending on time available. If you are able to continue on for several minutes, you may find yourself in a meditative state. That would be wonderful! And we'll talk more about meditation in Chapter 13.

Mindful breathing is a technique worth telling your family and friends about. I have shared it many times, and it works for everyone. My son has learned to use it during times in which he realizes his need (or when I request him) to redirect his silly, wiggly energy. Mindful breathing calms him and allows him to focus on the task at hand. He is then able to release his intense energy at a more appropriate time, usually during recess or other times outside.

Chapter 3 - Canned (Dead) Foods

Let's revisit this idea once again - if the majority of the food items you're feeding your family come pre-packaged, they may contain ingredients that are known, over time, to cause harm to the human body. And this time, in the case of canned foods, the "ingredient" I'd like to make you aware of isn't an actual ingredient at all, but rather a chemical used to line the cans before they are filled with product. This chemical is bisphenol-A, also known as BPA.
Perhaps you've heard of BPA in regards to water bottles. There was much press about BPA, a known endocrine disruptor, leaking into the water these toxic plastic bottles contained. In 2012, in an effort to "boost consumer confidence," the United States Federal Drug Administration (FDA) banned the substance from baby bottles and sippy cups.[5]
Unfortunately, BPA remains in other products, including canned goods.
The good news is that there are companies who have taken steps to remove BPA from their canned goods, and they do label them as such. If you continue to use canned goods, read the label and see if it says the lining is BPA-free. You may also consider switching to foods that come in glass or aseptic containers. At the very least, rinsing those canned goods that aren't already in a sauce of some sort, i.e. black beans, peas, or corn, will help to reduce the amount of BPA that is being consumed.

The other topic I wanted to touch on regarding canned foods is the fact that canned foods are "dead" foods. That is not to say they offer nothing nutritional. This isn't true. But they are lacking in some of the vitamins and all of the enzymes their truly fresh counterparts offer. I say truly fresh because sometimes the "fresh" produce I see at the local grocery stores looks like it would be better utilized by adding it to a compost bin, which means it, too, is no longer as nutritious as it once was. Yet again there is another alternative. Think frozen!

Chapter 4 - The "Dirty Dozen"

There is often debate as to whether or not organic produce is worth the extra expense. I would always argue it is, but as a single mom on a budget, I realize there are times when it's necessary to make choices. I'm going to share with you here a fantastic tool for deciding which fruits and veggies you must INSIST are organic in all their forms (i.e. fresh, juice, or sauce) and which ones contain little to no pesticide residue even though they were not grown using organic methods. Just to clarify, this tool relates entirely to pesticide levels. It does not speak to the nutritional value of these fruits and veggies nor how earth-friendly the methods were in which they were grown. Those are topics for those who wish to continue the debate in another arena.

The Environmental Working Group (EWG) is, in their own words, "a non-profit, non-partisan organization dedicated to protecting human health and the environment." A portion of their mission is "to empower people to live healthier lives in a healthier environment." Each year the EWG tests thousands of both domestic and imported fruits and vegetables to determine which ones are most contaminated and therefore the most potentially harmful to the health of you and your family. The results are published online, and they are most commonly referred to as the "Dirty Dozen." In fact, while the actual number may vary slightly each year, the complete list references nearly 50 fruits and vegetables. Those at the bottom of the list are referred to as the "Clean Fifteen."

Once you acknowledge your own level of comfort with pesticide residues on your food, you can use these lists and choose accordingly. For myself and my family, I will no longer purchase any fresh fruit or vegetables, nor any products made from the same, if they are an unfortunate member of the "Dirty Dozen." If we cannot find the item as organic, I won't buy any. There are always other options.

As we live in a climate where the growing season only lasts for 5-6 months at best, finding good quality organic produce can be a challenge, and I often find myself shopping from the "Clean Fifteen." The bright side of our cold winters is that soup is a wonderful, warm option for dinner, and there are plenty of root crops grown by our local, organic farmers that keep well in winter storage and make delicious soup!

You can view the "Dirty Dozen," the "Clean Fifteen," and the complete list for yourself at this website: www.ewg.org/foodnews. While you're there, I encourage you to "READ THE REPORT" for a full summary and further information about pesticides and how they may affect you and your children. Babies and young children, as they are not finished growing yet, do not have fully functional filtering systems, and they have the potential to be affected more by lower concentrations of pesticide residue. You will find within this summary a small report on the EWG's findings in baby food, as well.

I've quoted the key findings from the 2016 full summary below. Please be sure to check the website for annual updates (or sign up for email notifications) to keep yourself informed!

Regarding the “Dirty Dozen” -

- More than 98% of strawberry samples, peaches, nectarines, and apples tested positive for at least one pesticide residue.
- The average potato had more pesticides by weight than any other produce.
- A single grape sample and a sweet bell pepper sample contained 15 pesticides.
- Single samples of strawberries showed 17 different pesticides.

Regarding the "Clean Fifteen” -

- Avocados were the cleanest: only 1 percent of avocado samples showed any detectable pesticides.
- Some 89 percent of pineapples, 81 percent of papayas, 78 percent of mangoes, 73 percent of kiwi, and 62 percent of cantaloupes had no residues.
- No single fruit sample from the Clean Fifteen™ tested positive for more than 4 types of pesticides.
- Multiple pesticide residues are extremely rare on Clean Fifteen™ vegetables. Only 5.5 percent of Clean Fifteen samples had two or more pesticides.

With all of that said, here are the lists for 2016:

The "Dirty Dozen" Plus:

1. Strawberries
2. Apples
3. Nectarines
4. Peaches
5. Celery
6. Grapes
7. Cherries
8. Spinach
9. Tomatoes
10. Sweet Bell Peppers
11. Cherry Tomatoes
12. Cucumbers
    + Hot Peppers
    + Kale/Collard Greens

+ The Plus items were frequently found to be contaminated with insecticides toxic to the human nervous system.

The "Clean Fifteen":

1. Avocados
2. Sweet Corn (a small percent is genetically modified - choose organic to avoid)
3. Pineapples
4. Cabbage
5. Sweet Peas (Frozen)
6. Onions
7. Asparagus
8. Mangoes
9. Papayas (a small percent is genetically modified - choose organic to avoid)

10. Kiwi
11. Eggplant
12. Honeydew Melon
13. Grapefruit
14. Cantaloupe
15. Cauliflower

I have been truly grateful for the work of the Environmental Working Group since I first stumbled upon these lists. They allow me to do my very best when shopping for the foods I choose to feed my family. I hope you are able to enjoy a similar level of benefits, too!

Chapter 5 - Emotional Freedom Technique

"Your life is supposed to feel good to you." ~ Abraham-Hicks

There was a time not long ago that, if you had asked me what I knew about Emotional Freedom Technique (EFT), I would've shrugged my shoulders, shook my head, and said I knew nothing. And then one day I did know something, though I cannot remember how I first heard about EFT, also known as tapping. What I do remember thinking was what a strange concept it was and how weird I must look as I tried tapping for the first time. I am much less self-conscious now than I was then, but so far I still tend to do my tapping at home.

The modern concept of EFT incorporates tapping with your fingertips on a series of meridian points found on your body while speaking statements in conjunction with the tapping. This combination of activities will allow your body to release or de-energize the negative thing you are speaking about. The negative thing might be pain, a thought, a belief, or a fear. It might be something you are consciously aware of, or it might be something hidden in your subconscious mind which is presenting itself as a painful symptom or a negative habit or behavior.

The use of meridian points for healing dates back many centuries to ancient Chinese medicine. It was only during the 20th century that a connection was made between these same meridians and our

emotions. There are twelve main meridians, or energy channels, found in our bodies. The tapping technique that I use incorporates nine points. Each of these points is located where a meridian ends and is found just beneath the surface of the skin. As with most activities, there are other techniques available.
I first tried tapping to help shift the energy that I felt was preventing me from moving forward with my business plans, which included this book. I only dabbled in it, though, and I never made the time to tap during those moments when I felt the most stuck. It was when I just couldn't stay stuck any longer that I made the commitment to engage in an online tapping event. I was seeking release of unknown energy blocks and a level of engagement in my business that I had not been driven to experience before.

During this free event, I did no less than one tapping session each day. I would select the topic that my intuition lead me to choose. Often times I would do the tapping meditation at the end of my day, too. On several occasions, during both the sessions and the meditations, I could feel my energy channels open up. For me, this process of clearing can involve a lot of tears. Truth be told, I have come to love the sessions that include tears the most, because I have learned they are the ones that are the most life-altering. And as it turned out, it had been my self-worth that I had been working to heal. It is because of this healing that I am now free to fulfill my purpose in life, and I have chosen to begin that journey with this book.

To get started with tapping, you must first know where the meridian points are. I have included a diagram to help you learn their locations:

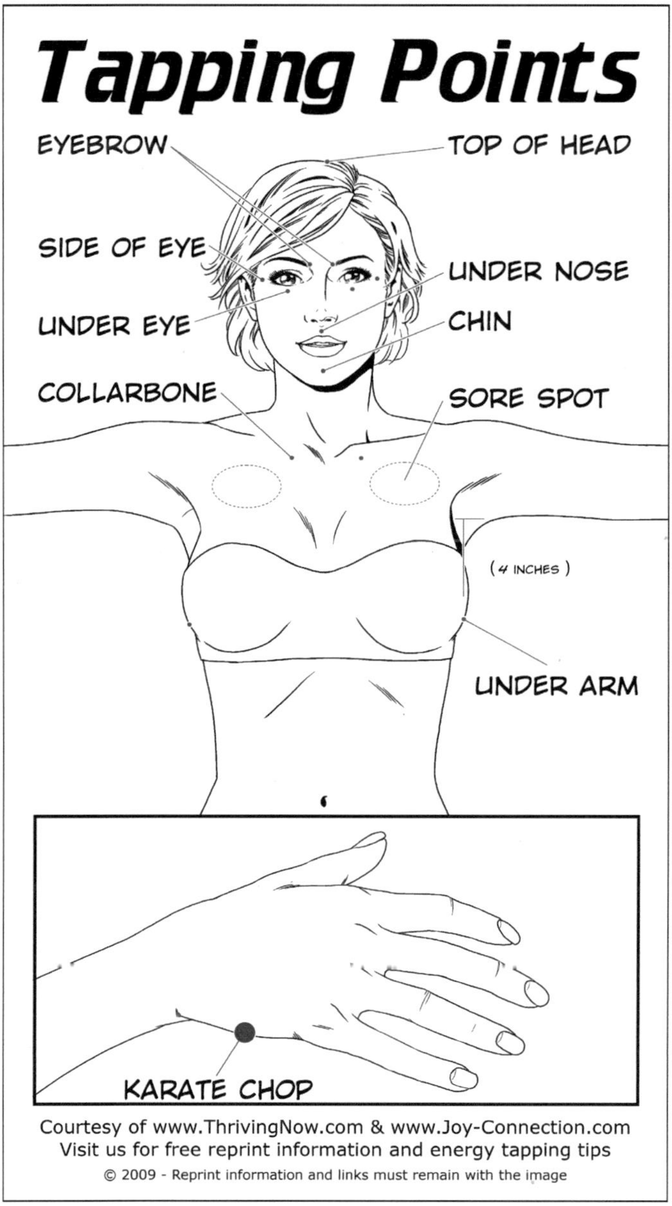

The tapping process itself begins with you defining what it is you wish to tap on. You might choose a particular pain or a more general sense of distress.

Once you have decided on your topic, you will need to rate the topic on a scale of 0 to 10; 10 being extreme intensity, and 0 being not noticeable at all. Next you will create your setup statement. Essentially, you only need to tweak the following sentence to make your topic of choice fit: "Even though I have/feel/am (insert topic here), I deeply and completely accept myself." With this statement, you will perform the tapping setup. Do so by saying your setup statement out loud while tapping with two or four fingertips on one of your two karate chop points. Repeat this sequence three times. After you've completed three rounds of saying your setup statement and tapping on your karate chop point, take a deep breath, first inhaling through your nose and then exhaling through your mouth.
Continue the tapping process by using two or four fingertips and gently tapping on each of the remaining eight points in this order:

1. Eyebrow
2. Side of eye
3. Under eye
4. Under nose
5. Chin
6. Collarbone
7. Under arm
8. Top of head

Tap at least 5-7 times while saying a simple reminder phrase at each point. For instance, if the topic of your setup statement is anxiety over an upcoming family gathering, you might use the phrase "this anxiety." As you did after completing your set up statements, take another deep breath. You have just completed your first round of tapping. Great job!

Take a moment to revisit the scale of intensity. Decide where your topic falls on the scale after one round of tapping. Ideally, the intensity will be lower than it was before you did the tapping. If you are still feeling any of that which you have chosen to tap on, do another full round of tapping. You may wish to alter your setup statement to include the reduction of your topic. Continuing along with the anxiety example, you might say "Even though I am still a little anxious about this upcoming family gathering, I deeply and completely accept myself," and your reminder phrase could be "a bit of anxiety." When you have completed this second round, tapping again on all nine points, take a deep breath!

To complete this tapping session, you will use phrases to increase the positive flow of energy into your body. A phrase to complete the example might be "I enjoy the feeling of calm I have now." Say this phrase while tapping at each of the eight points in the order they are listed. Once this is done, take a deep breath. Congratulate yourself for completing an entire session of tapping - nicely done!

Tapping is truly a unique tool to release negative emotions and rejuvenate your positive energy flow. It is free and, as long as you overlook HOW you look while you are doing it, tapping can be done anywhere. Feel free to join me at www.LiveWithVigor.com for a video session which will help bring clarity to your routine of tapping. Your emotional freedom is important! I believe you can do this!

Chapter 6 - Filter Your Water If ...

Consider the fact that, on average, 60% of your body is water. Water is a necessity for many of the life-sustaining functions that occur within your body each day. Again on average, you can only survive for three to five days without water. There is no doubt water is of great importance to all of us!

How much water should you be drinking each day? I don't have an exact answer for you. There isn't any science behind the old standard that says everyone should drink 8 - 8 ounce cups of water in a day's time. This isn't logical, anyway, as people do come in various sizes. It would stand to reason a larger being would require more water than a small one.

I've seen a second recommendation in which the amount of water consumed in a day's time should equal one-half of your body weight (measured in pounds) in ounces. For instance, if you weighed 140 pounds, you would drink 70 ounces of water each day to stay fully hydrated. I like this approach. It works well for me on an average day. Any time there are extremes, though, I find myself in need of more water. Extremes would include things like an intense workout, spending time outside in the heat of summer, or spending time in a sauna or a hot tub. All of these will cause your body to sweat and water loss will increase.

Another culprit when it comes to increased water loss is caffeine. Regular coffee, some teas, and some sodas contain caffeine. Chocolate, especially dark chocolate, is also a source of caffeine. Caffeine is a diuretic, which simply means it makes you urinate more often. That said, if you consume anything containing caffeine, plan to increase your water intake to compensate for the additional loss of water from your body.

While there is some truth in the idea that the color of your urine is a good indicator of how hydrated you are, or not, there are other reasons for a strong color concentration. Simply sleeping throughout the night results in a normal, stronger color in the morning. The best thing you can do when you wake up is drink 12-20 ounces of water to start bringing your body back to a fully hydrated state. Vitamins and some medications can alter urine color, too. In the end, definitely drink water when you are thirsty (some say if you're thirsty you've waited too long), and then drink any additional amount that allows you to feel comfortable throughout your day.

Now, let's review the water you choose to drink.

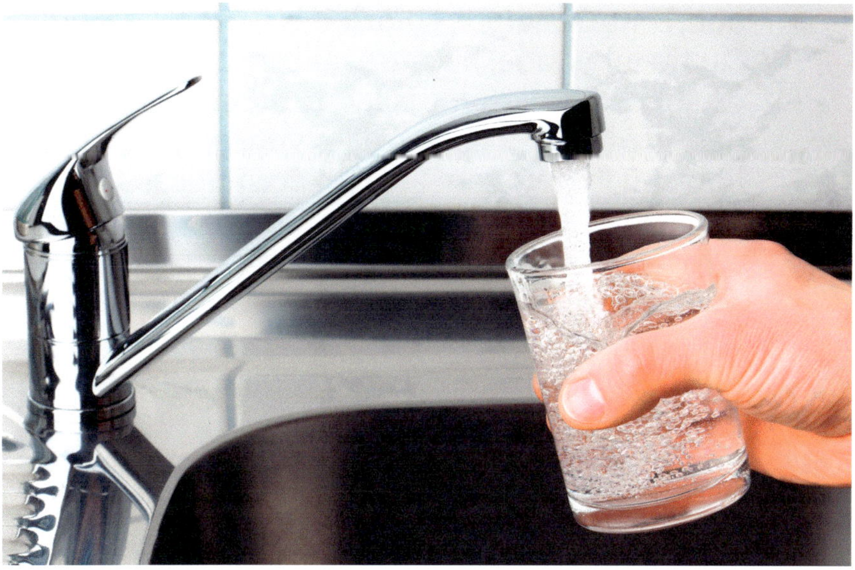

Are you drinking tap water from your local water treatment plant, or are you drinking well water that comes directly from the ground? If you're drinking bottled water, it either came from a water treatment plant or a groundwater source. I've seen figures that suggest up to 40% of bottled water is simply tap water from one city or another. Wherever your drinking water comes from, it's important to know a few things about all potential sources. Only then will you be able to make the best choice possible for your family.

Let's look at typical tap water first. Originally, water that comes to you via the public water supply was either surface water or ground water. Because government regulations require the water that comes into your home to meet certain safety standards, said water is treated to ensure you won't be exposed to high levels of bacteria that may cause illness. Chlorine is a common option used to accomplish this task. So, yay! No bacteria! Or maybe not. Unfortunately, chlorine is toxic to our bodies. On the plus side, because chlorine is a gas, it will dissipate if the water is left to sit uncovered for a period of time. There are varying opinions on just how much time is needed to accomplish this. A more efficient means of removing the chlorine (plus possible sediment and odor) is to use a carbon filter. These are very common and easy to find in a size just right for your needs.

As I type, I live about two city blocks away from our local water treatment plant. When I first moved into my house, it took only days before I smelled the waft of chlorine from my skin every time I stepped into the shower. It reminded me of my days as a member of the high school swim team and had the same side effects: my skin dried out, and I was itchy a lot of the time. I was NOT happy! The filter I invested in was big enough to service all of the water being used in my house, including my drinking water. I recall spending about $1500 USD. Every now and then I receive a phone call telling me it's time to replace the carbon, which I do without hesitation. Divided by the more than 17 years my filter has been in place, $1500 was a small price to pay for chlorine-free water!

Unfortunately, as I've learned since then, carbon filters cannot remove fluoride, another chemical commonly found in tap water. The main reason given for the addition of fluoride is that it helps prevent cavities. Unfortunately, the fluoride added in at water treatment plants is an industrial by-product that has not been purified and is not at all the same as the pharmaceutical grade of fluoride used in toothpaste[6]. There is good news in that not all communities are adding fluoride to their water supplies anymore, as there is much controversy surrounding this practice. The bottom line as I see it is that taken internally, fluoride is also toxic to your body.

There are very few methods to remove fluoride from tap water, and none of them are as inexpensive as the carbon filter that removes chlorine. I am most familiar with reverse osmosis, which is the filtering system I chose to have installed in our home several years ago. A reverse osmosis system does create a small increase in water usage, as it uses water beyond what will be consumed to clean itself. Some feel this is water waste, but with clean water being so crucial to good health, it works for me. For perspective, consider this: Most of us generate waste water when washing our dishes, our clothes, and our bodies, and those practices are accepted as normal. In any case, there are other options for removing fluoride, including water distillation, ionization, and ozonation.

Other contaminants which may or may not be present in your public water supply include prescription drugs, chemicals, and pesticides. How is this possible? Here's one example: When people don't know what to do with their unused and/or expired prescription drugs, they may decide to flush them down the toilet. This water is then returned via the sewer system to the water treatment plant and, once treated, this water is released back into the system. Eventually it makes its way to your kitchen faucet. No one really wants to be consuming someone else's prescription drugs. As a favor to all within your community, if this situation applies to someone you know, have them contact their local police force and ask if there is a "medicine take-back program" available to them. There is no filtering system within the public water supply that will remove any of these residues, and there are also no regulations against their presence in your water, at least not right now.

If your water supply comes from a well, you're not off the hook. Instead of the city monitoring bacteria counts, this responsibility belongs to you. If you live in an area of high agricultural activity, pesticide residues are also an increasingly alarming possibility. To the east of where I live, studies were done which unfortunately proved every well in that sandy area is now contaminated with not only previously recognized high levels of nitrates, but also low levels of insecticide residue. Homes for sale in these areas are required to have reverse osmosis systems installed. And the truth is, it's not only people who are at risk from these residues. Consider the bees as they fly about, only to find themselves being doused with irrigation water containing chemicals designed to kill insects. Bees are responsible for the pollination of about 30% of our food crops. Without pollination in these cases, fruits and vegetables cannot form, and there is no longer a viable crop to sell or eat.

What to do, what to do? First determine whether your water source does or does not contain potentially harmful substances. Use the reports made available by your public water source or seek out a water testing service near you. A Google search or your local county officials will be able to help you find one. Then, based on that information, decide what you wish to filter. If the filter option you desire doesn't fit into your budget right now, a temporary option is bottled water that has been filtered by reverse osmosis, ionization, or ozonation. Local to me, these are available for about $.80 USD per gallon. The information on the label of bottled water will tell you if it has been filtered in any of these ways.

As with most things, it's up to you to decide what is the best plan for you and your family. May you find power in putting your new knowledge to good use!

Chapter 7 - Growing Your Own Food

I currently earn my income as a grower. I oversee the fertility and troubleshooting components for the growing of hundreds of annual and perennial flower varieties within 2 acres of greenhouse space. I do the same for more than 150 acres of sand-grown sod. And last but not least, I spend time doing the same for several hundred acres of produce. I happen to have a gift, what I refer to as permanent plant files in my brain. Once information is installed there, it doesn't go away. I feel confident in my skills. I know I can figure out how to successfully grow anything!
I tell you this because there is an underlying truth to what I do: Growing plants is not rocket science. Relative to this conversation, growing food for your family IS an option! I believe you, too, (that's **who**!) can grow plants and, in particular, you can grow plants that will produce vegetables and fruits you can use to feed your family.
Perhaps you're questioning **why** you would want to!? I believe you might want to consider growing your own food, even if it's just one of something for now, for any or all of the following reasons:

1. No pesticide residues!
2. Incredible flavor!
3. Fun!
4. Mentally and physically therapeutic!
5. Time with your kids!
6. Continuing education!

7. Handy snacks and/or supper components!

"Okay, Debbie. I see there is value in growing food for my family. I live in an apartment complex, though, and I don't have any garden space. Just **where** do you think I am going to grow a plant?" Believe me when I say there are ALWAYS options (and they MUST include lots of sunshine!):

1. Some plants thrive in containers or hanging baskets on a deck, patio, or balcony that gets enough sunshine!
2. Partner up with a friend who does have garden space. Offer to trade your labor for fresh vegetables! If you don't have such a friend, ask someone in your neighborhood if they would be open to this idea.
3. Find a local church or community organization offering raised bed areas for people who wish to grow but don't have their own space.
4. Talk with your landlord about building a similar raised bed space on their property. In doing so, you will be able to maintain a neat appearance, and you won't need to purchase any large equipment, i.e. a rototiller.
5. Recent innovations using LED grow lights make growing indoors without any natural light at all VERY possible!

In general, gardens placed directly in the ground require more tools. They also require more kneeling, squatting, and bending, and while these make for great exercise, they aren't for everyone. Raised bed gardens and containers can offer bountiful produce

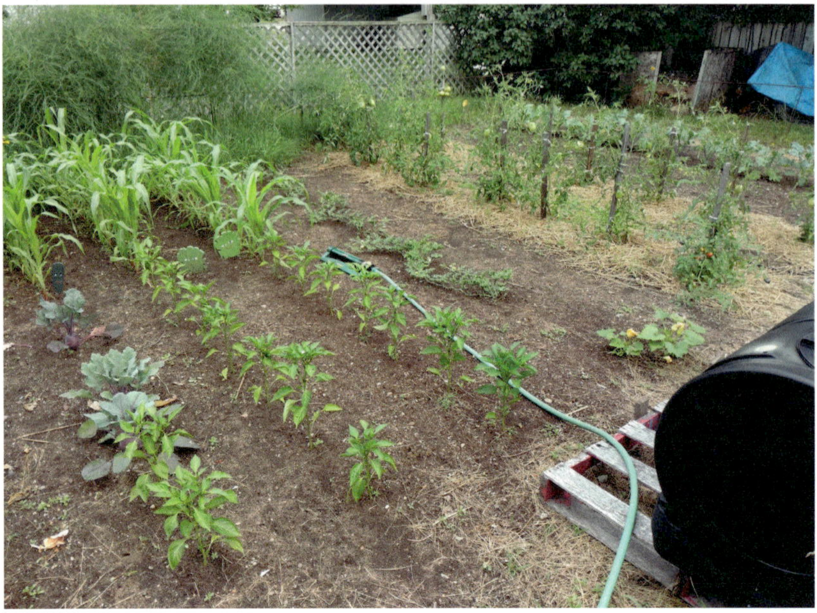

without the more intense workout it takes to prepare the ground for growing.

Myself, I have an in-ground garden. I enjoy the opportunity to exercise my body while I work in the dirt. I have a few perennial crops (rhubarb, asparagus, strawberries), too, and these would not come back each season if they were in a raised bed in my growing zone. The winters are too cold here and they would freeze out. My garden does require a fence or rabbits would take it over as their own. The fence also helps to redirect my children, their friends, and our dog while they are playing in the yard.

My sister and her husband, as another example, have invested their time in building raised bed gardens. They have a small backyard and two very active dogs, so they decided this was the best option for them. They live in a mountainous region of western United States and, because of their typically very short growing season and frequent chilly nights, they took their raised beds a step further and added hoops across the top so they would be able to draw frost covers over the beds at night without damaging the growing plants underneath.

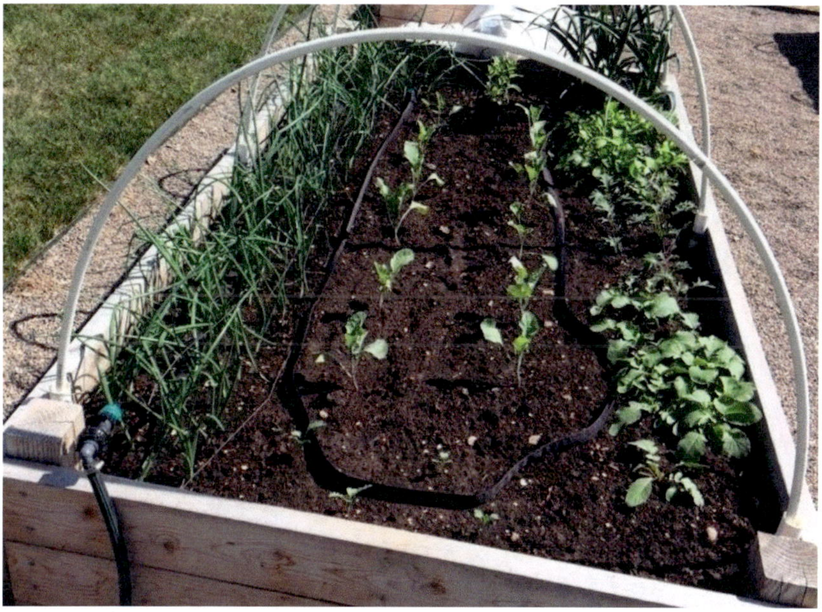

To note, they harvested so many vegetables from these four beds they were able to freeze enough to supply themselves with organic vegetables throughout the winter months. This is possible for you, too!

What will you need to begin your growing project? Wherever you have decided to give growing your own food a try, be it container, garden, or raised bed, know this: **The soil you are using is KEY to the outcome of your project**! Honestly, you could grow your plants on top of an asphalt driveway if you

give your plants the proper soil and moisture. True story.
Produce will grow best in soil that drains well and has a sufficient amount of composted (broken down - i.e. no longer recognizable as leaves) organic matter to provide quality nutrients the plants will need to flourish. I would recommend seeking organic products. This would include bags of potting mix if you are going to be using containers and bags of organic fertilizer if you are going to be working within either the natural ground or a raised bed in your yard. Regarding the soil needed to fill raised beds, it is most likely you will source this from a local landscape/nursery business. They typically offer gardening soil in bulk, which means no plastic packaging waste and a lower cost for you.
I mentioned the necessity of good drainage. If the soil in your yard seems to remain wet for days or even weeks after a 1/2" rainfall, this suggests either your soil has been compacted by too much heavy traffic (perhaps during the construction of your house) or your soil is clay-based. Clay-based soils will have to be *heavily* amended to achieve proper drainage. The better option here might be to consider the raised beds. In any case, if you are purchasing soil for any situation, you might first check the drainage quality by putting a small amount of soil in a small container with holes in the bottom and then pouring what would amount to an inch of water over the top of the soil. Watch to see how long it takes for the water to drain through. It should happen within just a few minutes. If it takes hours, don't use the soil.
Give some consideration to whether you prefer to start with seeds or plants. By selecting seeds, you have complete control over which varieties to plant. I

love this part! There are tastier varieties out there than are typically available at your local greenhouse or garden center. I would recommend making sure to select seed that is certified non-GMO and, if possible, organic. In doing so, you will be supporting farms that recognize the environmental importance of how we choose to grow food. I have my favorite seed sources listed under "Resources and Links" at my website: www.LiveWithVigor.com.

I live in a northern climate, which means my growing season isn't long enough to produce certain foods were I to start them from a seed in my garden. This includes peppers of any variety and tomatoes. For these vegetables, I either start my seeds indoors at the appropriate time listed in the directions on the seed packet, or I buy my plants. If you are able to locate a local plant sale or a greenhouse or garden center that sells organic transplants, this would be an option that not only supports your gardening efforts but also sustainable practices that promote good care of our earth.

Planting either seeds or transplants in your growing space is a great activity to share with your kids! My son's favorite seeds to plant are sugar snap peas. I know he loves to eat the finished product, but I am also certain he prefers planting pea seeds because of their size. The only difference between a fresh pea and one used for planting is the one for planting is dry and wrinkled. They are both similar in size, and that size happens to be an easy one for smaller fingers to grasp and plant.

There is great value in allowing kids to help with the growing process. They may take ownership and help with the chores necessary to grow the vegetables. You may also find they are more willing to try eating different vegetables because they have taken these vegetables on as their own. Gardening with kids can be an excellent experience. I encourage you to share this time with your kids and find out for yourself.

I mentioned earlier, where you have chosen to grow your vegetables will dictate how many tools you are going to need. Containers, the smallest option, will require nothing more than making sure there are drain holes at the bottom and perhaps a small trellis or garden stakes if you are growing vining crops like cucumbers, squash, or tomatoes. Beyond that, all of your work can be done with your hands.

Raised beds, once installed, will only require a trowel and a rake. You can consider these as hand tools or as full-length options. In-ground gardens will require the full-length options. Also for in-ground gardens, my must-have tool if you wish to beat the weeds in a hurry - the hula hoe! It skims the ground just under the surface, and when the weeds are tiny, it separates the top of the weed from its roots, causing it to die. Because it stays just under the surface of the soil, it doesn't introduce a new weed seed crop that would then germinate and grow all over again. In my opinion, the hula hoe is the best gardening invention ever!

If you decide you would like one for yourself, you might find it useful to know the hula hoe is also called a stirrup hoe. If you aren't able to locate one at your local hardware store or gardening center, you will be able to find them from various online sources. A simple Google search will help you locate these sources.

The other ingredient you must supply for success is adequate water. In general, no less than an inch of water per week is necessary to produce a good vegetable crop. If this water doesn't come to you in the form of rain, you will need to supplement by using either a watering can or a sprinkler attached to a hose. If you do supplement, **the KEY is to water deep and less often!** Roots are lazy. They will only move as far as they have to for water. If the water goes deep, so will the roots, and their going deep is important for successful vegetable gardening. This is true of any plant, and it is a good growing practice no matter what you are growing.

When are you going to have the greatest success in growing your vegetables? A good rule of thumb for most vegetables is to wait to plant until two weeks after the last average frost in the spring for your area. Of course, if you live in an area which never receives frost, your growing schedule will be during the more temperate months of the season, as it is tough to keep things growing when the temperatures rise higher than 85 degrees Fahrenheit during the day.

For a more in-depth gardening manual, sign up at my website, www.LiveWithVigor.com, to be notified when Gardening 102 becomes available. You can do this! I believe in you!

Chapter 8 - Hemp for Breakfast ... huh?

Personally, I am not fond of eating any kind of meat more than once or twice each week. It slows down my digestive system, and I simply don't feel my very best. Over time, I have researched and found other suitable options to ensure I have adequate protein in my diet. One of the options I've found is hemp protein. For me, hemp turned out to be a great protein option for breakfast.

Hemp is a plant. There is more than one variety of hemp, as is the case with many plants. The hemp plant which is the source of this protein is not the same as the one that is used as a drug. Hemp is grown as an annual crop, which means it is a sustainable, renewable resource. It offers huge potential for both its fibers and its food value. It is unfortunate that it is also illegal to grow this non-THC (not marijuana) form here in the United States. The hemp products that I source come from Canada. I list my favorite source under the "Resources & Links" tab at my website: www.LiveWithVigor.com. The edible portions of hemp include the leaves and the seeds. Hemp seeds have a mild, nutty flavor. According to the fine folks at Nutiva, "The hemp seed balance of Omega 3 to 6 fats is the perfect proportion for human dietary needs." I like to add these seeds to salads and tomato soup.

More often than the seeds, though, I use hemp protein powder. I like to make breakfast smoothies with it. There are recipes on each package of protein

I buy, but quite simply all it takes is your favorite liquid source and a favorite fruit or two, plus the protein. I use almond milk, blueberries, a banana, and spinach, plus the powder. I have also been known to add in a bit of pure maple syrup for sweetness.

What I like best about using hemp as a protein source is that it contains all nine essential amino acids, making it a complete plant protein. Few plant foods can boast this truth. These essentials are vital for good health and, because the human body cannot produce these amino acids on its own, eating all nine of them often is very important. Hemp protein also happens to be easy to digest. Along with the protein, hemp offers lots of dietary fiber, and when you combine these two things with a few simple ingredients, you have a breakfast that leaves you feeling satisfied well into the morning.

Chapter 9 - Intuition & Food Choices

Intuition can be defined as "the ability to understand something immediately, without the need for conscious reasoning." It is something we are born with, something we all have inside of us and, indeed, it is a great indication that WE DO KNOW what is best for ourselves.

I believe children live in this state of knowing but, as they grow, they are inundated with the beliefs and suggestions of others, and by the time they (we) reach adulthood, they (we) are no longer in touch with the inner knowing that is vital and necessary for them (us) to become their (our) best selves. When we do not allow our intuition to be our ally and our guide, we can do no more than live out the lives that others have knowingly or unknowingly set before us. From where I sit today, I am telling you that a life dictated by others is merely a life of mediocrity. It cannot be a life filled with passion and love and joy if it doesn't come from within YOU!

Intuition often comes into play when making decisions. Some decisions require little to no intuition at all. For instance, what you will need to buy at the grocery store is dependent on what you choose to eat and how many of those things you still have in your refrigerator, freezer, or pantry. On the other hand, intuition is very useful in learning to make healthier food choices. As you practice strengthening your intuitive skills, you will learn to "hear" what your body has to say after you feed it the foods which you have chosen to prepare meals with.

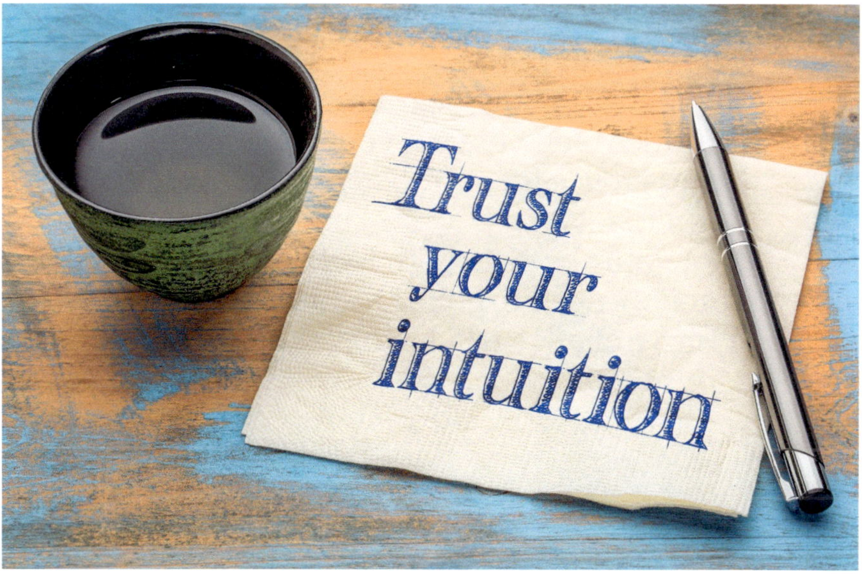

I have several thoughts on how you can strengthen your intuition regarding food choices:

1. Listen to food thoughts that enter your mind as you move through the grocery store.
2. Skip the multi-tasking and put your entire focus on your shopping experience.
3. Note how you feel when you observe what others are putting into their shopping carts.
4. Allow yourself time to reflect on your food thoughts and how you are feeling as you prepare a meal.
5. Allow yourself time to reflect on how your body is feeling immediately after you have eaten.
6. Note how your body is functioning several hours after you have eaten.

7. Note your high/low energy levels throughout the day.
8. Listen to and record any additional food thoughts that enter your mind.

As you continue to learn more about making healthier food choices, your innate sense of what is a better choice for your body will blossom. You will begin to feel the power in making food choices which allow your body to both look and perform at its best. You only need to continue, even in baby steps, and positive change will be inevitable!

Chapter 10 - Juicing

My sister sent me a juicer as a gift long before I would actually start juicing. I do admit that it sat on my counter for quite some time before I actually used it. I still have this *Jack LaLanne Power Juicer*, a well-marketed centrifugal juicer which is still available today.

The centrifugal juicer is the most basic of at least three types of juicers available. There are many details to juicing worth noting which will help you make your decision as to whether or not juicing is something you would like to incorporate into your healthy habits. Before I write about them, however, I would like to start with why it's worth the effort to juice something in the first place. Why not simply eat the fruits and vegetables in their whole form (which is also a healthy option)?

Juicing separates the nutrients, including vitamins, minerals, and enzymes, of the fruit or vegetable from the fiber it contains. This leaves those nutrients in a ready-to-absorb form, and your body is able to take them and distribute them directly to the cells of your body. There is no need for your body to digest and then break down the food first. The marketing phrase for this is "nutrition at a cellular level."

It is true that you are what you eat, and if you "build" your body with inferior building supplies, somewhere down the road your body may begin to fail you. Consider the story of the three little pigs. It was the pig who used brick and mortar for his foundation whose house was able to withstand outside forces and remain strong, while those houses built by his brothers using weaker materials of straw and sticks did not remain standing long at all! If your body is in need of repair, and you wish to repair it as fast as possible, getting the very best nutrition to your cells via juicing is an excellent way to do this! One important point to remember - if you decide to juice, you may wish to consider your juice as THE choice for either breakfast, lunch, or dinner. Fresh juice likely contains more calories than the original fruit or veggie it was made from, as the juicer is more effective at "digesting" those items than your body is. If you add extra calories into your current eating routine, your weight may increase. When I do juice, I find it works best as breakfast.

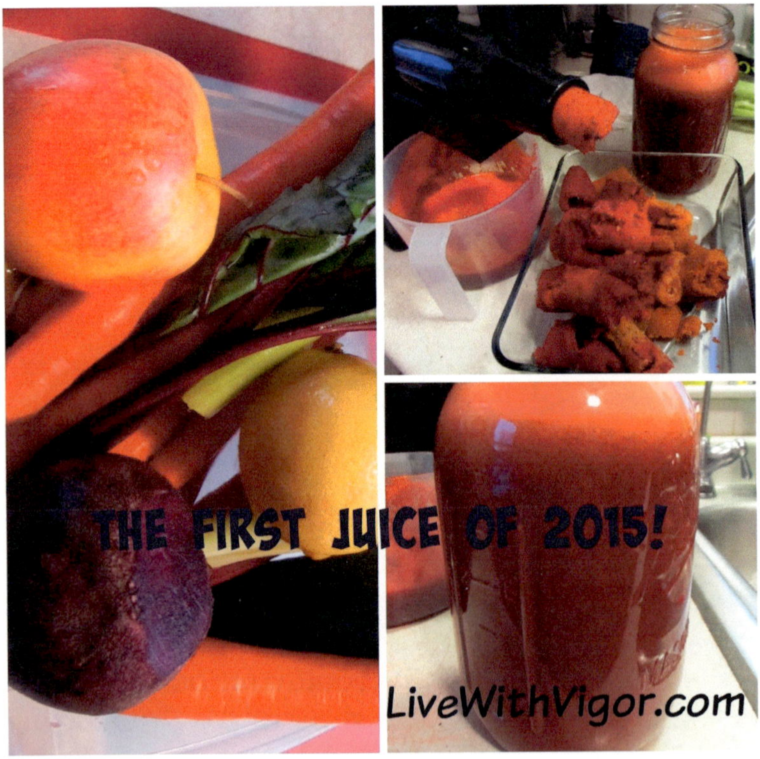

Now, on to the details regarding choice of juicers:
A centrifugal (a.k.a. basket) juicer is typically the least expensive type available, which makes it a great choice if you would like to try juicing without making a significant investment. They are definitely the most readily available as well, as you can usually find one within any department store that stocks small kitchen appliances.

Centrifugal juicers work by shredding the fruits and veggies as they are fed into the chute and then spinning these shredded pieces to extract the juice. This process is not the most efficient juicing process, but it is easy to use and also easy to clean. There are two potential drawbacks to using this juicer. The first is that to receive the greatest benefits from the juice it must be consumed immediately after juicing is done. The centrifugal action creates friction and heat which in turn begin to oxidize and break down the quality of the juice soon after the process is complete. The second is this type of juicer will not work for greens, including wheatgrass, spinach, and kale.

A masticating (a.k.a. single gear) juicer is the first of two options if you wish to add greens to your juice. I currently have access to a Champion model of this type of juicer. My observation is it takes more overall time to complete the juicing process with this masticating juicer. The vegetables must be chopped into smaller pieces, as the chute feeding the produce into the juicer is not as large as that of my centrifugal juicer. Also because the mechanism by which it juices is slower, it takes a few extra minutes before I am able to drink the fresh juice.

That said, this slower speed means less heat is generated as the vegetables and fruits are being crushed to extract their juice instead of being shredded and spun. This minimizes oxidation and preserves valuable nutrients, which in turn offers you the option to store the juice for a day or two in your refrigerator.

Masticating juicers are more expensive than centrifugal juicers. They typically fall in the middle of the pack as far as price is concerned. You may find masticating juicers for sale in your town if there is an organic or natural foods store there. Otherwise, there are several models available to you via online outlets. In case it is important to you, they are much heavier than centrifugal juicers, and they take up more counter top space as well.

The third type of juicer, and the second of the two that will juice greens, is the triturating (a.k.a. twin gear) juicer. This type of juicer works similar to the masticating type. It is slower in operation, and it produces no heat, so the juice it produces can be stored in the refrigerator for the greatest amount of time. It is supposed to be THE most efficient juicer in terms of juice extraction because it uses two augers instead of one. It also happens to be the most expensive type of juicer. As with the masticating juicer, you may have to shop online to find one. I have never had a triturating juicer myself. Based on the recommendations of those who have, though, Green Star models are the favorite choice in this category.

If you decide to do some online browsing of juicers, you may notice both the masticating and triturating juicers have additional features that allow them to make things like nut butters, sorbet, pasta, and baby food. Consider these features as you consider how much you will use your juicer and how much you would like to spend on one.

My thoughts regarding the produce I use in my juicer include the following:

1. If the produce I am using was purchased in a store, I ALWAYS use a produce wash to clean them first. I also peel cucumbers and carrots.
2. If the produce I am using came from my garden, I rinse them to be sure they don't have any dirt on them. I never peel anything. I know the fruits and veggies I grow in my yard are free of food-grade wax and toxic pesticides.

When the time comes to clean your juicer, it is important to know cleaning is much easier when you do it right after juicing. Another observation you might find helpful is that over time, white juicers will develop stains in the areas where the juice concentrates. If these stains are not acceptable to you, consider buying a dark-colored juicer.
When I use the masticating juicer, my favorite containers for storage are canning jars. Glass is BPA-free, easy to keep clean, and doesn't stain, and the juice inside is always beautiful to see. Of course, there are plenty of other options available. I have the jars in my basement, though, so the cost is perfect for me!

Chapter 11 - Know Where Your Food Comes From

One of my favorite t-shirts is orange in color and has the words “Who’s Your Farmer?” across the back. In fact, I had it on the day I wrote this chapter. How appropriate, because in this chapter I will share with you my thoughts on why I feel it’s important to know where your food comes from.

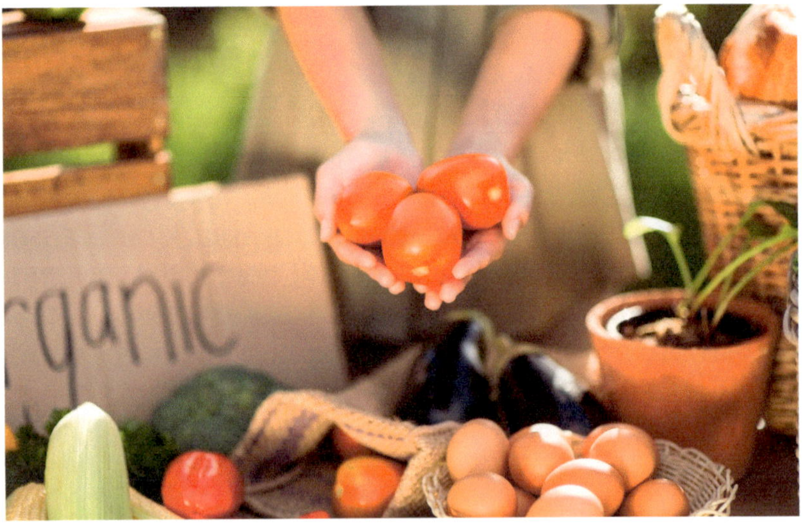

First and foremost for me is this: Knowing where your food comes from is the easiest way to ensure you are eating clean, whole foods. By clean I mean without pesticide residues, chemical ingredients, or genetic modifications. I believe clean, whole foods are the foundation of good health. As local food campaigns are becoming more and more prevalent across the entire United States, options for finding whole foods from trustworthy sources are many:

1. **Farmer's Markets** can be found in even the smallest communities during the local growing season. Fresh produce is found in abundance at these markets, and most of the time this produce is sold by the families that are growing it. As you stroll through the market, take time to talk with the people under the tents and behind the tables. Ask them if they grow their veggies without chemicals. Ask them if the animals they raise are free of growth hormones and antibiotics, or if they make sure the animals do not eat any genetically modified feed. If they sell products made from the produce they grow (i.e. jam or salsa), read the ingredients labels to see if their ingredient choices meet with your approval. As you continue to reach out to the growers, you will develop connections that will keep you coming back to the same tables week after week. Before you know it, you will have a good relationship with your local farmers, and you will feel confident in knowing the food you are feeding your family is as fresh and full of nutrients as possible!

2. **Community Supported Agriculture (CSA) Farms** continue to make their produce available to families who wish to buy a share in the farm's harvest at the beginning of the growing season. Typically, each week a full share of fresh produce is no less than one-half bushel of produce. That can be a lot for families who are just getting used to using fresh, whole foods in their meal preparation, so often times half shares are available, too. In lieu of purchasing a share, many CSA farms offer a limited number of worker shares. In return for a specified number of hours volunteered each week at the farm,

workers will take home their share of produce without having to pay for it. This partnership ensures all of the field work, harvest, and packing are done in a timely manner and rewards the workers with an abundance of fresh produce. I have done this myself for two growing seasons, and in doing so I was exposed to a wonderful array of heirloom varieties of vegetables whose flavor surpassed anything found in typical grocery stores. I met some very interesting people who shared new food recipes as well as new methods of preserving those foods so they keep into the winter months. Honestly, I enjoyed this time working in return for a share of organic vegetables, and I felt a superior level of satisfaction that came with knowing I was bringing home the highest quality food available to feed my family. A good resource for locating either of these first two options is available at www.LocalHarvest.org.

3. **Grocery stores with local food programs** are becoming more common. In my community, one of the grocery stores has implemented local foods into their produce department. Pictures of the farmers, along with a small description of the farms, can be found throughout the department. It is my opinion that these offerings aren't quite as fresh as buying them directly from the farmer, but they are a better choice than fruits and veggies that were picked green and ripened in a warehouse because they have better flavor.

4. **Online markets** are an option I use when I am looking for a quality source of food that cannot be grown in my area. Specifically, I have located online markets for both raw almonds and raw walnuts. In each case, these are family-owned farms who communicate with me personally each time I place

an order. I feel confident in the production methods, which are explained on their respective websites. Each time I place an order I know who I am supporting, exactly what I will be receiving, and precisely where it came from. Visit the "Resources and Links" tab at my website for links to those markets I am currently supporting: www.LiveWithVigor.com.

A secondary benefit to choosing foods grown by your local farmers is doing your part to leave behind a much smaller carbon footprint. A carbon footprint is the measure of impact a process has upon the earth's environment in terms of carbon dioxide (pollution) output. This means it makes good environmental sense to buy carrots grown near to you instead of those that need to be shipped even several hundred miles. For instance, here in Wisconsin, USA, if I decide to buy carrots grown in California, I know they have traveled approximately two thousand miles to get here. Consider that good fuel mileage for a semi truck is nine miles per gallon. Simple math shows that 200 gallons of fuel would be used to move those carrots 1800 miles. That's a whole lot of fuel burned in the engine of the truck that made the delivery! How big is your carbon footprint?

Chapter 12 - Laugh Often!

"Always laugh when you can. It's cheap medicine." ~ Lord Byron

"A day without laughter is a day wasted." ~ Charlie Chaplin

"I love people who make me laugh. I honestly think it's the thing I like most, to laugh. It cures a multitude of ills. It's probably the most important thing in a person." ~ Audrey Hepburn

It seems these benefits of laughter have been generally recognized for centuries:

1. Relief from negative stress
2. Strengthened immune system
3. Improved blood circulation
4. Increased mental function
5. Enhanced well-being

In-depth studies of laughter have shown laughing to be as important to your daily regimen as proper sleep, sound nutrition, and regular exercise. Essentially, laughing acts as exercise. It stretches muscles, sends oxygen to body tissues, and it releases neurochemicals that make you feel good! All of these benefits appear to be in direct correlation to how much we laugh - the more we laugh, the more benefits we receive. And the truth is, who doesn't want their levels of feel-good to be as high as possible? I know I am ALWAYS up for more laughter!

What to do, then, to laugh more? Here are a few ideas for you:

1. Play with your (or someone else's) kids! Kids don't feel the same pressures that stem from responsibility as adults do, and they don't need to be reminded to loosen up. Consider this as your reminder: Loosen up! Go play, and remember to let your beautiful laughter sound out loud and clear!
2. Hang out with friends who love to laugh, too, and hang out with them more often! Statistics show we laugh more when we are in social situations... a LOT more! So, use your phone, Skype, or some other form of communication and invite these funny friends to be a part of your day or your week or your month, even if only for an hour or two! Just do it.
3. Create a plan to inject humor and, hopefully, laughter into your normally boring or mundane work activities. The neat thing about laughter is that it's contagious, and the likelihood is if you need more laughter in your life, so do your coworkers. Feel free to substitute "work" with any other area of your life that needs more laughter.
4. Look at yourself in the mirror and start laughing. I'm not kidding. It works.
5. Type "images of laughing hysterically" into your search bar and have a look at what shows up. Allow your smile to form and your laughter to come out. Remember, it will make you feel better, and you will be glad you did!

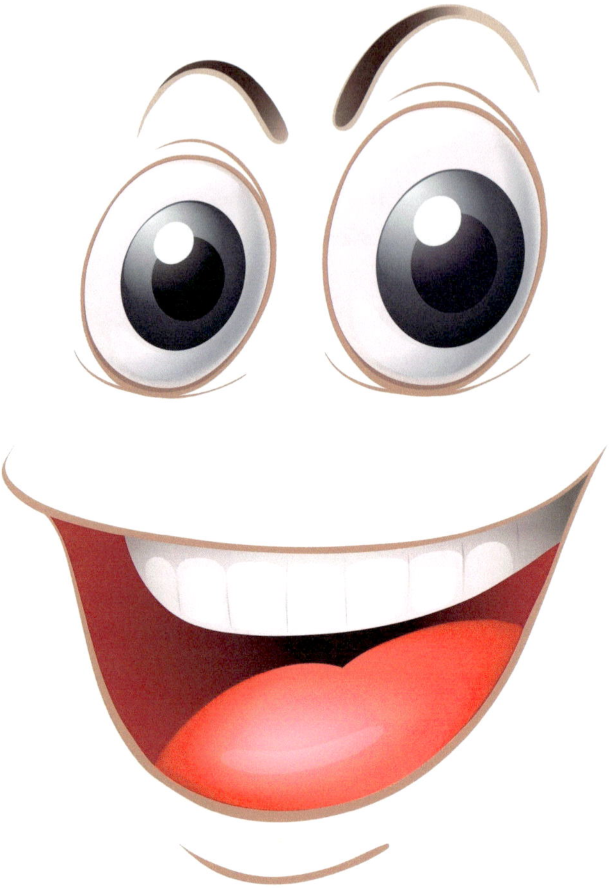

There is suggestion among researchers that laughter on your own, while it does indeed benefit your body, does not offer as equally powerful effects as those experienced when shared with family and friends. While interesting, and a good reason for surrounding yourself with positive people, don't let it keep you from laughing out loud on your own, often!

Chapter 13 - Meditate - Find the Quiet

I have been meditating on and off for several years. I began my meditation practice with a 21-day challenge offered by the Chopra Center. Twenty one days is the minimum number of days it takes to create a new habit, and the thought is that after you successfully complete the challenge you will then both want and be able to incorporate meditation into your daily life. The number of proven benefits is increasing every year, so committing to 15-20 minutes of meditation each day is, in my opinion, a very valuable use of time. My truth is I meditate more often than not now, but I am still not meditating every day. I believe the benefits are important enough, though, that I am on task to make meditation a daily habit.
In a nutshell, the following are some of the known benefits of meditation:

1. Increased focus
2. Increased creativity
3. Increased memory
4. Increased compassion
5. Increased productivity
6. Reduced anxiety
7. Reduced stress
8. Reduced pain
9. Reduced depression
10. Emotional balance

There are many different types of meditation, and as I would suggest with most things, after you have the chance to give several of them a try, choose the type you feel the greatest connection to. Choose the one in which you are able to quiet your mind the most, feel your greatest connection to Source energy, and hear the answers to any questions you have asked.
I believe the easiest way to get started is with a guided meditation. These meditation segments will be, as the name suggests, guided by someone. Each segment will begin with a short discussion of its topic followed by music or sound designed to help you slow the thoughts passing through your mind. In my opinion, the objective isn't to silence your mind, but rather to become an observer of the thoughts that pass through, reserving any judgment or emotion that you may have associated with them at other times.
I still take part in the Chopra Center 21-day challenges. Deepak Chopra is the guide for these meditations. Another favorite meditation leader of mine is davidji. They are both easy to locate online. You can also find a very large archive containing many different types of meditations at www.WinterFeastForTheSoul.com. I have specifically shared the "Young People" section with my daughter. I believe there is great value in giving the gift of self-awareness to our children, and I truly appreciate this wonderful resource which helps me do so.
There is no right or wrong way to sit for meditation. Simply make sure you are comfortable. I find an upright position works best, but I have also been laying flat on my back. If you are very tired, laying down will likely end up in your falling asleep and,

while sleep is a good thing, you won't receive the benefits of meditation if you do.

There are different schools of thought on when to meditate. Using the acronym RPM helps you to remember the morning process - rise, pee, and meditate. Late in your day, before you prepare to go to bed is another option. During both of these time periods your brain is in such a state as to allow the shift in awareness. Should you decide to try to meditate during the busiest portions of your day, you may have difficulty finding the quiet you are seeking. But then again, perhaps it will be exactly what you were needing.

Chapter 14 - Nuts

Nuts are considered an excellent snacking choice by many, and rightfully so. Nuts contain healthy fats including omega-3s. These fats are important for both heart and brain health. Nuts are packed with protein and, as a snack, this protein, plus the fiber found in nuts, goes a long way towards keeping hunger pains at bay. Nuts also contain varying amounts of antioxidants, vitamins, and minerals, all of which are needed by your body to stay healthy. A proper portion for snacking would be about one handful, the hand belonging to the person eating the nuts, of course.

What types of nuts make the best snacking choices? Almonds and walnuts often top the list. Other quality nut choices include cashews, hazelnuts, Brazil nuts, and pistachios. Macadamia, pecan, and pine nuts finish out the list. In case you're wondering what happened to peanuts, well, peanuts aren't really nuts at all. They are a member of the legume family, and as such are related to peas and beans. They have a few peculiarities which make them the topic of a separate conversation.

The best quality nuts would be fresh, organic, and raw. Nuts that are old or improperly stored can go rancid. A rancid nut has an unpleasant odor and should be thrown away. To increase the shelf life of nuts, keep them in sealed containers and place them in either the refrigerator or the freezer.

Organic nuts will be free of pesticide residues. Raw nuts will contain all of the goodness, including vitamins and enzymes, they were grown with. There is an unfortunate exception here that everyone has the right to know. That exception is almonds grown in the United States.

In 2007, the U.S. government passed a law that required almonds grown in the United States to be pasteurized before they could be sold. This law was created after two incidents in which a salmonella outbreak was traced back to California almond crops. No deaths were reported from either of these outbreaks. What does this mean to you?

If you're purchasing U.S. almonds from any storefront here in the United States and the package claims they are natural and/or raw, they cannot be both, and they just might not be either. They have been pasteurized by one of two treatments. The most detrimental of these treatments is fumigation using a gas called propylene oxide (PPO). PPO was once used as racing fuel, and it has since been banned from the racing circuit because it was found to be carcinogenic. Yet somehow our government has deemed it okay to use on the conventional almond supply.

The second option for pasteurization is steam. Heating the almonds in this way will kill any bacteria present on the almonds. It will also kill the enzymes in the almond, effectively eliminating any truly raw properties it once had. Steam pasteurization is the only allowable treatment for organic almonds, and I believe it is the best of the two options. If the almonds you buy are not organic, you will definitely be able to find companies out there that are choosing the steam option. It might be wise to make a phone call or send an email to the customer service department of your particular brand of almonds and ask them which type of pasteurization they are currently using.

Because of two exclusions in this law that requires pasteurization, there is a relatively unknown, yet far better (in my humble opinion), third option. Almond farmers are allowed to sell unpasteurized, truly raw almonds directly from their farms or roadside stands in quantities of less than 100 pounds. Some farmers have been clever enough to create online roadside stands from which to sell their almonds. This is the option I choose for my family. You will find the farms I choose to use listed on my website: www.LiveWithVigor.com.

Chapter 15 - Oils and Other Fats on Your Plate

I have met many people who have fallen victim to claims that eating fat will make you fat. The truth, however, is that healthy fats will NOT make you fat. You only need be aware of the types of fats found within our food supply, and then you will be able to choose the healthy ones and eat them without concern. Before identifying some "good" and "bad" fats, I believe it may help if you understand why every human body needs fat in the first place.

- Our bodies use the fats we eat as their energy source for the many functions they perform each and every day to keep us alive. That said, if we eat more than our bodies need, the excess will indeed be stored for future use.
- Fats are necessary for the proper functioning of our brains and nervous system. The myelin wrapped around our nerve cells allow the nerves to send important electrical messages to other areas of the body. Did you know the brain is said to be made up of about 60 percent fat? Improper fat consumption may leave you in a mental fog, with the inability to concentrate, or having difficulty remembering things.
- Our bodies need the essential fatty acids we eat for proper growth, development, and cell

function. The body cannot produce these essential fatty acids on its own.

- Fat-soluble vitamins A, D, E, and K require the fats we eat to transport them to the areas of our bodies where they are needed.
- Fat is necessary for our bodies to form the hormones required to regulate many body processes. It also plays a major role in healthy hair, nails, and skin.

The first type of fats on "the list" are **trans fats**, the type you should ***avoid*** eating. While there are small amounts of trans fats found naturally in a few foods we may eat, the majority of these fats are artificially created through a process known as hydrogenation. They are commonly found in fast foods, fried foods, and commercially processed foods like cookies, crackers, and snack foods. These fats are also found in margarine and shortenings. You will recognize them in the ingredients list as hydrogenated or partially hydrogenated vegetable oils.

The problem with trans fats is how they negatively affect cholesterol levels in our bodies. Instead of promoting a healthy cholesterol ratio, trans fats raise the "bad" cholesterol (LDL) and lower the "good" cholesterol (HDL) at the same time. Maintaining a healthy cholesterol ratio is very important to good heart health!

The second type of fats are **saturated fats**. Saturated fats are found in animal products including butter, cheese, milk, ice cream, and meats. They are also found in a few tropical plant oils including palm and coconut.

There are two schools of thought about saturated fats. The first is that all saturated fats are bad and you should avoid them. The concern here is the potential for increased cholesterol levels, which in turn would increase one's risk of having a heart attack. Instead, I agree with the second school of thought that says specifically selected foods containing saturated fats offer health benefits that override the potential for increased cholesterol levels. I feel it is important to note, however, the foods I eat which contain saturated fats are by no means the greater percentage of my food intake. I simply enjoy them from time to time without concern.

If you recall, I mentioned selecting those foods containing saturated fats with care. For instance, if I am going to eat eggs, I make sure they either come from a friend who allows her chickens to roam or else I buy eggs produced by pastured chickens at the local natural food store. If I eat meat, it is usually venison or local pasture-raised (grass-fed) beef, chicken, or pork. The organic milk and butter I buy is also produced from pasture-raised cows. I would expect by now you are seeing this picture more clearly. The source of the foods you eat matters.

The final type of fats I will mention here are the **unsaturated fats**. These fats can be mono or polyunsaturated. In either case, these fats will not raise cholesterol levels and, in fact, they may indeed help to lower cholesterol levels that are too high. Unsaturated fats are found in greatest concentrations in nuts including almonds, hazelnuts, pecans, and walnuts, avocados, seeds including pumpkin, sesame, and flax, and fatty fish including tuna and salmon. They are also found in vegetable oils including canola, soybean, olive, and peanut. Unfortunately, there are again conflicting viewpoints on whether vegetable oils are healthy or not. In fact, because of some research I did for this chapter, I am now having to decide if I will continue using grape seed oil for cooking or not. This is a little technical, but it turns out the polyunsaturated fat in grape seed oil is damaged by heat and causes free radicals to form. So, I am leaning towards not, though I don't really use it all that often anyway.

I plan to stick with organic coconut oil for my stir-fries. I will continue to use organic extra virgin olive oil for things that don't require heat, such as salad dressing. Because life tends to be busy, occasionally it's just easier to buy salad dressing. I look for one with a base of organic canola oil. I already mentioned I use organic grass-fed butter. If we do use oil for the occasional batch of brownies or classroom cupcakes, I will likely find an organic sunflower oil. I don't prefer to buy anything that contains soybean oil, organic or not.

In the end, ALL oils are processed, and they are not the best choice for adding fat to your eating routine. Processed oils are never as healthy as eating the whole foods the oils came from in the first place. Be brave and experiment a little! Here is one experiment I tried: Because I'm always seeking healthier choices, instead of an oil-based salad dressing, I tried a mashed avocado on my salad. It was delicious! Fresh-squeezed lemon juice gives this an extra punch! I will continue to experiment to find fats that work best in our eating schedule while at the same time leaving my kids and I feeling mentally alert and full of energy!

Nutrition facts labels are found on the majority of food items sold in grocery stores here in the United States. At this time, these labels are required to identify both saturated and trans fat quantities per serving of the labeled product. Any mention of unsaturated fats is currently provided on a voluntary basis. I would like to offer a helpful hint to figure out how many unsaturated (healthy) fats are in your food choices if this information is not volunteered on the label.

Total fat grams are listed as a percentage near the top of any label. Just under this will be the percentages for grams of saturated and trans fats. Add these two percentages together and subtract from the total fat percentage. To determine if the remaining number is the percentage of unsaturated fat found in one serving of the product you are looking at, take a quick look at the milligrams of cholesterol on the label. Convert these milligrams to grams by moving the (figurative) decimal point three places to the left. If this number is now greater than one, subtract it before considering the final percentage as unsaturated fat.

In the end, remember that fats are necessary for good health. Choose foods with healthy fats instead of those labeled as fat free. Use the information you've learned above to make healthier fat choices for your family. And congratulate yourself on adding another rock solid layer to your foundation for a healthier life!

Chapter 16 - Protein Sources - Where Did That Cow Grow Up?

Protein is one of three macronutrients essential to proper functioning of your body. (The other two are carbohydrates and fat.) These macronutrients provide the calories, or energy, we need for growth, metabolism, and other body functions. The fact that protein is a macronutrient means not only is it necessary, it is necessary in relatively large quantities when compared to vitamins and minerals, which are micronutrients.

Protein is a component of every cell in your body. Your hair and nails are almost entirely made up of protein. If they're not in great shape, perhaps you might review your protein intake to be sure it is sufficient.

The amino acids contained in protein are the building blocks of your body's bones, muscles, cartilage, skin, and blood. As well, protein is a component of several body chemicals, including enzymes and hormones.

Protein helps to build and repair tissues. After a strength training workout, I like to eat at least 10-12 grams of protein, which for me seems to benefit muscle repair and make for a quick recovery. In case you didn't know, building muscle is one of the best ways to help with weight loss, if doing so is a goal of yours. Muscle burns more calories than fat.

I've mentioned two of my favorite plant proteins in chapters 8 and 17 in this book. Both hemp and quinoa are complete proteins and are suitable replacements for protein sourced from animals. That said, I do eat meat from time to time. The caveat is that, as with anything I eat, I am very particular about where this meat and all other animal products come from.

Why might it matter where the meat you consume comes from? From my perspective, there are three potential things to consider:

1. What did your food eat before you ate it?
2. How environmentally friendly was the process of raising the animal?
3. Were the animals treated ethically?

There are two very distinct sides to this conversation. The first reflects a cleaner, kinder, more natural approach to raising animals for their food products, which likely results in a safer, healthier food product for your family. The second involves what are referred to as confined animal feedlot operations (CAFOs), also known as factory farms. CAFOs continue to earn themselves a bad reputation, raising animals in inhumane, unsanitary conditions and causing irreparable pollution of our water and air.

With the first approach, animals are raised in pastures of grass and other annual and perennial plants. These animals have plenty of fresh air and sunshine. Their waste is scattered and subject to degradation by nature's sun, rain, and critters. Because these animals are able to move freely in open air, their risk of illness is small.

In the middle of this discussion lies a gray area where the two styles of production intermingle just a bit. Some pasture-raised animals are fed grain (usually corn) shortly before they are to be slaughtered. This speeds up weight gain which puts the farmer's meat on the market just a bit sooner than would otherwise happen. On the plus side, this diet of grain is usually strictly vegetarian and made of only plant foods.

The second approach, the CAFO, exists solely for the quickest production possible. As the name suggests, these CAFO animals are confined, and they cannot experience the benefits of sunshine and fresh air. Add to this the fact their bodies are not designed to eat grain, and they experience much higher rates of illness. To prevent the illness that does occur from spreading through the entire feedlot, these animals are all given antibiotics.

Feedlot animals grow fat faster. To ensure this, their food is supplemented with growth hormones. Their diets of grain are also supplemented with animal by-products, which I believe is an unhealthy and potentially dangerous practice. You may recall mad cow disease and then wonder why a vegetarian animal is being forced to eat a non-vegetarian diet of rejected animal parts and pieces. Realize it is possible for infected animal by-products to contaminate the meats you choose to feed your family. There is nothing pleasant about that possibility in my opinion!

Waste generated at a CAFO is filled with everything that was first fed and/or given to the animals. It is generated in very large quantities, and the stench in the air is overwhelming and can be noticed several miles away from the feedlot. The waste becomes hazardous as it is spread on farm fields and drains

into surrounding watersheds. Heavy rains close beaches when high levels of e-coli are washed in from neighboring CAFOs. Water pollution has also caused severe algal growth and fish kill. In no way is this waste part of a sustainable ecosystem.
Interestingly enough, many of the same unhealthy aspects of the CAFOs can be applied to fish farms. Farmed fish are being fed corn and soy products, which are non-fish foods. Reduced nutritional levels of one of the key components and why fish are eaten in the first place - omega-3 fats - is the result of this practice. Some reports[7] show the reduction for farmed salmon is nearly 50%! Farmed fish are also held in close confinement and experience a similar, significant rise in disease potential, not only to themselves but to any wild fish swimming past their confinement pens. The practice of farming fish also causes pollution of nearby waters, and the risk of damaging fragile coastal ecosystems is very real.
In any case, once you are in the know, you will be able to make an educated choice as to which protein sources you choose and where you would like them to come from. My logic says it stands to reason that if I choose the cleaner, kinder approach for any meats we may use, I will do the same for any products that come from animals but are not the animals themselves, such as eggs, yogurt, and cheese. In fact, it would be more typical within my diet to use these products, especially free-range, organic eggs, rather than the animals themselves. I also use organic milk from pasture-raised cows to make milk kefir, which we then use as a base for smoothies.

How much protein you consume in a day is the secondary topic of this chapter, one that is also open for interpretation. The United States Department of Agriculture (USDA) MyPlate[8] program suggests 5 to 6-1/2 ounces of protein per day for adults, dependent upon your age and whether you're male or female. Using an average 7 grams of protein in 1 ounce of cooked meat, this would equate to 35-45 grams of protein each day. The number of grams will actually vary significantly when you start comparing strictly vegan options. Hummus, for instance, is only 1.2 grams per ounce. In another example, 8 ounces of almond milk contains only 2 grams of protein.

If it is true that the human body does best with .8 grams of protein per kilogram of body weight, then I feel the USDA range is a bit low. I feel it is definitely low for anyone on a regular workout schedule, and something to this effect is stated on the USDA Protein Food Groups chart[9].

If you're wondering how many kilograms you weigh so you are able to determine how much protein might be the right amount for you, I've got you covered! Take your weight in pounds and divide that number by 2.2. Then you can multiply the resulting number by .8 to find a reasonable number of grams of protein to consume each day. (You can actually also multiply your weight in pounds by .36 and achieve a similar number.) This formula is referred to as the Dietary Reference Intake, and the resulting number is the recommended grams of protein each day for sedentary adults.

As you work to adjust the amount of protein in your diet, keep this in mind: If you are increasing the amount of protein you eat, you may find you snack less often and/or need fewer carbohydrates because the protein will keep you feeling full for a longer period of time.

Chapter 17 - Quinoa

Let's begin this chapter with, well, how in the world to say quinoa. Quinoa spelled out phonetically is keen-wah. It is native to Bolivia and, interestingly enough, it is related to Swiss chard, spinach, and beets. Unlike its relatives, though, quinoa is a powerhouse when it comes to protein! One cup of cooked quinoa contains 8 grams of protein. Quinoa, like hemp, contains all 9 essential amino acids, making it another complete plant protein. If you recall, these 9 amino acids are absolutely important to good health, and you do need to eat them because the human body does not produce them by itself. In addition to protein, that same cup of cooked quinoa has 5 grams of fiber and provides generous quantities of iron, magnesium, folate, and more of those heart-healthy omega-3 fatty acids everyone is talking about!

Quinoa is sometimes referred to as an ancient grain. This means it hasn't changed in thousands of years. It is not hybridized or genetically modified in any way. I know there are some who will be relieved to learn quinoa is a gluten-free grain. It is available in three basic varieties - red, white, and black. My kids are partial to white quinoa. It has a softer texture than the red. They think the red is too crunchy. Sometimes I do, too. We haven't found any black quinoa to try as of my writing this book.

Quinoa is delicious as a stand-alone part of any meal. It is technically not a cereal grain (cereal grains are true grasses), but don't let that stop you from using it as a breakfast option. My son prefers it with just a bit of organic grass fed butter and organic tamari sauce. If you're used to the standard American triad on your plate, which consists of a meat, some form of potato, and a cooked vegetable, consider using quinoa as a replacement for both the meat and potato. Add to that a fresh salad and call it a meal once each week.

There are many yummy quinoa salad options out there, too. In fact, you can resource a few in the "From Our Fans!" link on my website: www.LiveWithVigor.com. Feel free to submit quick, simple recipes that you consider delicious. I would love to add them to the collection!

As far as taste, quinoa has a rather mild, slightly nutty flavor. This is what makes it such an easy swap for noodles and rice. We like to use it as a stir-fry base, replacing the rice. When it comes to making supper, I am often pressed for time between work and the evening's soccer practice or other activity. In these moments, quinoa saves the day because it cooks up in less than 20 minutes. Yay!

We have also used quinoa noodles to replace wheat noodles in our meals. They taste good. My advice would be to follow the cooking instructions so you don't overcook them. Also, they have a tendency to develop a dry texture if refrigerated and not mixed into something after cooking. Keep in mind that noodles are made from flour. That said, if you're looking for a gluten-free flour alternative, consider quinoa flour.

Chapter 18 - Raw Foods

For many years, if someone asked me for one simple tip to begin making healthier eating choices, I have said they might consider eating something raw with every meal. I still suggest this today. I believe, even if you use fast food (I sure hope you don't!) as your family's main source of meals, when raw foods are added in to the mix, they will, at the very least, provide living enzymes which will go a long way towards helping to digest the other "food-like" substances found at fast food restaurants.

Raw foods - what are they? The raw food list generally consists of fruits, veggies, nuts, seeds, and sprouted grains. Depending on your choice of foods, raw can also include eggs, dairy, meat and fish. I have no experience with the latter options, though, and I will not be making any recommendations for or against them.

Raw foods will remain "raw" as long as they do not reach temperatures higher than 118 degrees Fahrenheit. This is the temperature above which enzymes and certain vitamins and minerals will be lost and the "living" benefits of raw food no longer exist. Raw food eating habits help your body access much higher quantities of these nutrients.

Some will say you should be eating an 80:20 ratio of raw to cooked foods. This would be an overwhelming task for all but the most committed. My feeling in regards to any food choice is that you eat and then assess how your body is feeling an hour, or even a day, later. Are you feeling fired up and full of energy? Or are you feeling sluggish and as though you could

use a nap? Your body is very capable of giving you direction in regards to what you choose to nourish it with.
Raw foods will definitely give you more energy. And I will suggest to you, the more of them you eat, the more you will notice the difference. Around the time when I was low on the totem pole of self-worth, I was compelled to eat a primarily raw, vegan diet. I was contemplating divorce (see Chapter 25) and I found that despite all of the negative stress I was experiencing, I had never known such high energy levels as I did then. In keeping things honest, I was a stay-at-home mom then and I had more hours in a day for the preparations required for such an involved eating regimen. Worth the time invested? Absolutely! Am I still eating this way? No. Several years back I had to return to the workforce and I have yet to manage my time to allow for this to happen. My plan now is for financial freedom so I can hire someone to help in my kitchen!
It's okay to start with baby steps. Add a piece of fruit to your breakfast plate. Have some fresh veggie sticks with your lunch. Eat a handful of raw nuts as an afternoon snack. Consider a salad with supper. Keep preparations simple. Truly, start with small changes, take moments to notice how you are feeling, and continue on as your body suggests what is best for you. You can do this! I believe in you!

Chapter 19 - Sunshine (Without Sunscreen)

When I was a kid, it was because of my love for horses that I learned where the vitamin D our bodies require comes from. I had been selected to be a member of the Horse Bowl team. We were a team of three preparing to pit our horse knowledge against that of another team. The materials we studied contained a picture of a horse standing in a pasture on a sunny day. The horse was eating grass. Now, I'm no longer sure which vitamins the horse was obtaining as it ate the grass, though if I took an educated guess I would say vitamin A. I know for sure, though, the letters coming down from the sun and onto the horse were Ds.. D-D-D-D-D-D-D.

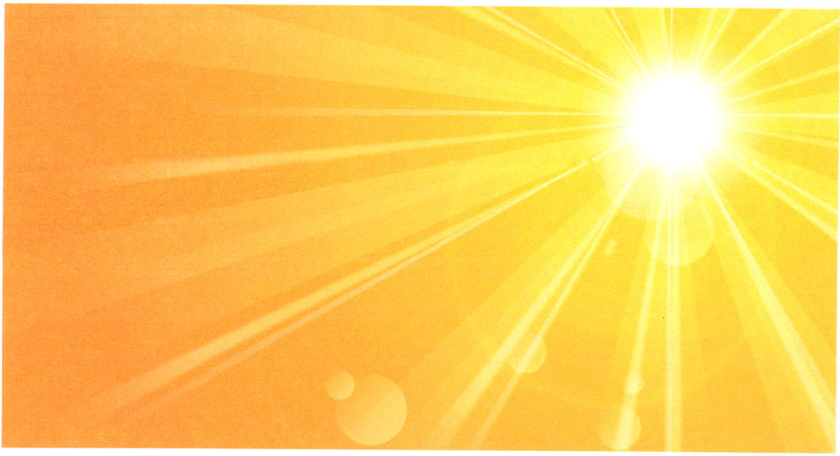

It is true. The best way for your body to manufacture proper levels of vitamin D is to soak up some beautiful sunshine! Sunshine! It takes at least 15-20

minutes of exposure to the sun, across 40% of one's body, at least three or four times each week, for a person's skin to absorb enough of the proper rays of sunshine to make appropriate amounts of vitamin D for themselves.

There are conditions for this to work:

- NO sunscreen!
- You must be outside, not sitting or standing in a sunny window!
- If you have a dark complexion, it will take more time in the sun to absorb enough rays. You may consider daily exposure or increasing the number of minutes exposed. It is important to be mindful so you don't end up with a burn.
- If you're in the northern hemisphere and it's winter (November - March), you may need supplemental vitamin D or an appropriate tanning bed. You'll want to find one with an electronic ballast that puts out UVB radiation.[10]

At this point, I may have left you wondering what vitamin D does for your body. The most important thing to know is that it is crucial for proper immune function. A strong immune system goes a long way towards good health for you and your family! And the best form of vitamin D is D3, the one that your skin is able to produce, for free, from sunshine! With that said, go play with your kids! Hang out with them while they swing, slide, and kick soccer balls in your yard! Go for a walk! Have your picnic lunch in a sunny spot instead of the shade, at least while it's not too hot for comfort outside!

On days where sun exposure will be much longer than is necessary for vitamin D, then take precautions to prevent sunburn. My recommendations include hats to shade your face and sun-protective clothing. If you choose to use a sunscreen, consider using this guide to help you in selecting a safer product: *http://www.ewg.org/sunscreen/*. If the link is no longer a viable one, simply do an internet search for "Environmental Working Group sunscreen" (no quotation marks when you're searching) and you will find reliable help.

Chapter 20 - Take Your Time

My role as a single mom comes with a long to-do list similar to that of any parent. Without a doubt, I have come to realize I will never complete the list. That doesn't mean I didn't used to try. I am a woman. Ha! Who better than a woman to be great at multi-tasking? After all, our brains are hard-wired for this! Not! It turns out that multi-tasking is neither a real thing, nor a good thing.

While it is true that a woman's brain happens to be hard-wired to make them better at multi-tasking than men, there isn't a human, male or female, who can actually perform multiple tasks simultaneously, unless you include those that are rather automatic, like breathing, walking, or chewing gum. All any of us can really do is switch back and forth between these tasks. This switching back and forth is a lot like what a computer processor does, except we fail to keep track of all necessary information like the computer does. Instead, we are likely to lose information as we switch back and forth, leaving us with less than desirable results on all accounts. As an example, for this reason, I don't write unless my kids are otherwise occupied for at least 2-3 hours. My train of thought derails if I am interrupted and I find it difficult to retrieve those thoughts. In any case, writing doesn't work when my kids are nearby.

Perhaps you've tried talking on the phone while following a new recipe you were making for supper? If you couldn't remember whether you'd added a particular ingredient, it may not taste quite as good as it might have had you focused exclusively on making supper. Or maybe your child has asked to watch TV while they do their homework, insisting they are ready for their quiz in math tomorrow. This appears to be a parental no-brainer, but I know it happens. If your child's grades are less than you know they are capable of, help them find a way to focus on one task at time.

Despite the fact we are never actually multi-tasking, science has proved when we do attempt to accomplish multiple tasks at the same time, we are actually less efficient than if we chose to complete one task before starting another. In writing this chapter, I came across a study that showed we will arrive at our destination later than otherwise if we are talking on a cell phone while driving a vehicle. The study fails to mention safety aspects, but it appears to me as if there are some to consider.

I do wonder how many of us actually need research to tell us about this inefficiency. I, like many, am left feeling distressed and somehow more frazzled if I try to accomplish too many things at one time. Hence my decision to take my time! I have found the benefits of taking my time include the following:

- I am able to maximize each moment of my day when I do one thing at a time.
- I am aware of the details. I remember them better.
- I am mindful of my surroundings.
- I appreciate the details.
- I give proper attention to those whom I have interactions and/or conversations with.
- I notice the flavors of the foods I eat, and it's likely I eat less of them.

- Daydreaming and the creative process that follows come easier.

Clear your mind and tackle your to-do list one task at a time. Life becomes more manageable when you do. I promise.

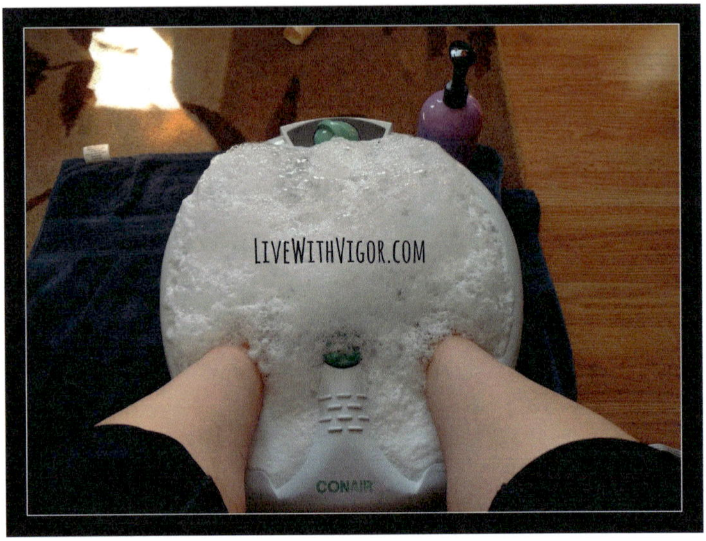

"All is well, and you will never get it done. Life is supposed to be fun. No one is taking score of any kind, and if you will stop taking score so much, you will feel a whole lot better — and as you feel a whole lot better, more of the things that you want right now will flow to you. You will never be in a place where all of the things that you are wanting will be satisfied right now, or then you could be complete — and you never can be. This incomplete place that you stand is the best place that you could be. You are right on track, right on schedule. Everything is unfolding perfectly. All is really well. Have fun. Have fun. Have fun. Have fun!" ~ Abraham-Hicks

Chapter 21 - Unique is a Wonderful Thing!

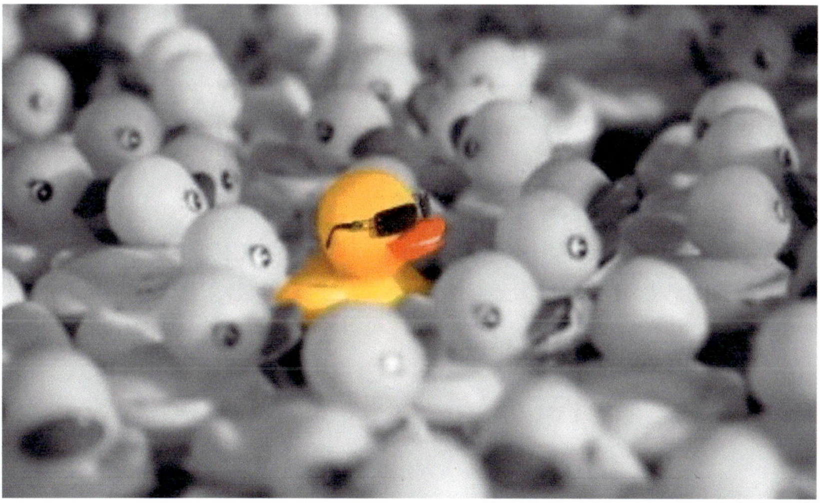

Thanks to David Levine at IntegrateIdeas.com for this stand-out picture!

"Having a low opinion of yourself is not 'modesty.' It's self-destruction. Holding your uniqueness in high regard is not 'egotism.' It's a necessary precondition to happiness and success." ~ Bobbe Sommer

"So you're a little weird? Work it! A little different? OWN it! Better to be a nerd than one of the herd!" ~ Mandy Hale

Consider the quotes above reflections of my opinion on how important it is to be true to yourself, letting those qualities that make you unique shine through.

I realize this can be easier said than done. There is more than a small amount of pressure from others to conform.

From the time we are small children, we are expected to behave in ways our parents would prefer. I remember a time when I was old enough to be a member of the school band. I wanted to play drums. I was told drums were not an option. I did play clarinet, but it was never my favorite instrument. To this day, I am still captivated by drum lines and drum solos!

Conformity is present in the school system, too. Students in schools across America are required to take standardized tests during the school year. There is pressure to perform well, and these tests cannot compensate for kids who are intelligent but don't test well. Yet there is no second option.

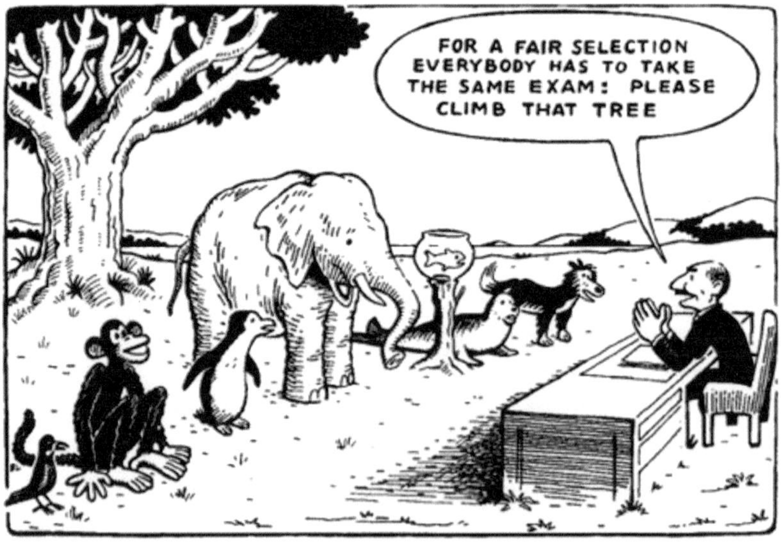

As adults, if we choose to believe what mainstream media tells us, we should all be wearing the latest fashions while we follow questionable nutritional guidelines, and then when we're ailing we won't hesitate to visit our medical doctors often so they can prescribe to us antidotes that cause other problems we didn't even know existed.

The truth for me is this: We are not here on this earth to conform to someone else's standards. We were born with an innate knowing of what is right and good for ourselves. So many of us were never encouraged to let these unique qualities shine through. The pressures of conforming to society's will has caused many people to lose touch with this inner knowing.

No matter, though. Today is a new day, and if you haven't already, it's time to start recognizing those things that are important to YOU! What makes you giddy with excitement? What brings you great joy? What leaves you feeling peaceful at the end of each day?

Every day, in EVERY situation, we gather information. If we allow it, the information we gather serves to help us learn what it is that drives us to become better human beings, what it is that calls us to greater service, and what it is that allows us to know happiness regardless of what others may say or do to try and bring us down.

Will you allow it? I believe only in doing so will you be able to become your best self and know true happiness.

P.S. My son, when choosing which area of music he would most like to learn in his first year of middle school, chose band, and when he was asked which instrument he would like to play, he said drums. I was grinning from ear to ear! I said yes!

"Be who YOU are and say what YOU feel because those who mind don't matter, and those who matter don't mind." ~ Dr. Seuss

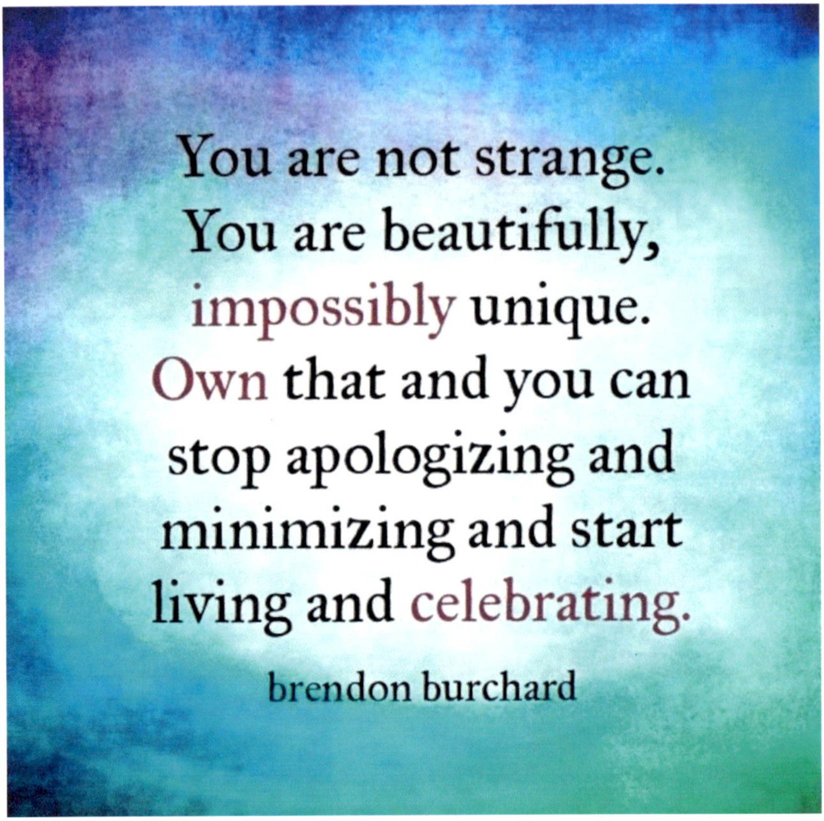

Chapter 22 - Vitamin B12

While many vitamins are important to the various functions your body must perform every day, I choose to focus on B12 because as critical as it is, vitamin B12 is mostly only available in animal foods including meat, fish, poultry, eggs, and dairy. I want to make sure you're aware of this availability if you choose plant-based eating habits.
Vitamin B12 has many functions which help to keep our bodies healthy. Here is the short list of the three main functions and how low levels of B12 will affect our bodies:

1. Vitamin B12 is necessary for the production of red blood cells. A shortage of red blood cells can lead to anemia, leaving your body feeling weak and fatigued and unable to properly fight infection.
2. Vitamin B12 is needed for the normal function of nerve cells as well as to manufacture myelin, the material surrounding the nerve cells that assists with neural transmission. Improper transmissions can affect appetite, sleep, memory, learning, mood, and behavior.
3. Vitamin B12 is required for the replication of our DNA cells. Without this replication process, our bodies cannot generate new, healthy cells. Symptoms of reduced replication would be similar to the effects of aging on our

bodies, including changes in memory, intestinal malfunctions, and wrinkles.

When my eating habits were entirely vegan, I added two things to my eating routine to ensure I was receiving adequate amounts of vitamin B12. The first of these was a sublingual vitamin B12 supplement. Sublingual means this vitamin is applied under the tongue. The one I used came in a small spray bottle. There is also a tablet form available. Both are very easy to use. In my opinion, there are two important things to look for when sourcing any vitamin supplement:

- Source of the supplement ingredients - My first option will always be an organic, non-GMO source. This includes any coating or capsule that surrounds the supplement. At the very least, I would make sure the supplement is non-GMO and made from a high quality source. I would use the internet or talk with a knowledgeable employee at a natural foods store to do my research.
- Absorption reviews - Many of the supplements advertised in mainstream media have very poor absorption rates. Again, I would use the internet to research the best absorption rates amongst available options. It is worth realizing that no supplement will have an absorption rate equal to that of a whole food vitamin source. All components of a whole food source work together to deliver the vitamins to your body in the most effective way possible.

The second thing I added to my eating routine was nutritional yeast. Nutritional yeast resembles powdered cheese. It does have a flavor that reminds me of cheese, as well, though if you're a true cheese aficionado, nutritional yeast likely will not meet your expectations! Despite this fact, I like it on top of pasta and spaghetti sauce. I also include it as one of six ingredients in the green drink powder I make. It is important to know that not all nutritional yeasts are created equal. If you decide to give it a try, be sure to read the nutrition label to make sure the one you choose actually contains vitamin B12.

The recommended daily amount of vitamin B12 is less than 3 micrograms, which is a very tiny amount. Also, vitamin B12 is stored in the liver for rather long periods of time. I have seen estimates ranging from 5 to 20 years. If your eating habits have included animal products, you will not have to worry about a deficiency in vitamin B12 unless you choose strict, plant-based eating habits over a long period of time. In this case, make the decision to supplement with either of the above options, and all will be well!

Chapter 23 - Whole Foods (aka Boxed Foods, Begone!)

When you consider the different ways you are able to create healthier eating habits, it is important to know that the more whole foods you choose to use, the healthier your habits will be. As with other topics relating to healthy eating, there is some confusion as to what constitutes whole food. I will share my thoughts. You decide which of them work best for you and your family.

Whole foods - consider them a product of nature rather than a product of the food manufacturing industry. In other words, whole foods are not processed or refined, and they will not contain chemical additives or other artificial substances. They will contain all of the nutrients and fiber they were grown with. Some examples of whole foods include a haddock fillet, raw milk, eggs, apples, lettuce, black beans, and peanuts that remain in their shell.

The easiest way to identify a whole food at the grocery store is to read the ingredient label. There will only be one ingredient, and if there is no label, you will know for sure what you hold in your hands is indeed a whole food.

That said, there are times when a whole food is more readily enjoyed after it is processed. Technically, as soon as a whole food has been chopped, frozen, or cooked, it becomes a processed food. In the case of those black beans, it will be difficult to enjoy them unless they have been processed (cooked) to make them soft enough to eat. The same is true for other foods such as the haddock, the eggs, and other foods including rice, lentils, and quinoa. (I know, some people do choose to eat raw fish and raw eggs.) After cooking, all of these foods remain intact and contain the majority of the components they were grown with, excepting those nutrients which are lost during the cooking process. If you are considering a processed food, turn again to the ingredient label. The best processed foods will contain very few additional ingredients, and it is likely you will be able to actually identify all of them!

One processed food we like to keep on hand is peanut butter. I buy an organic creamy version, and the only ingredient on the label is organic roasted peanuts. Another favorite of mine is raw almond butter. Again, there is only one ingredient on the label - organic raw almonds. I buy this one less often, though, as it is less available in my area and also more expensive. My kids prefer the peanut butter anyway.

Continuing along this path, the next steps in food choices would begin to lead you back to the more refined, less healthy ones. These foods are found primarily in boxes, cans, and bags. Their ingredient list is often long, and this list may contain many words that you don't recognize and cannot pronounce. My words of advice about choosing refined foods - use them sparingly, and when you do, be sure to buy organic. The organic label will ensure the worst chemical additives and preservatives are not present in the labeled product. It will also ensure the foods you are choosing have not been genetically modified.

An honest example - my kids, like most, love macaroni and cheese from time to time. I make sure to choose a brand that uses organic wheat and/or rice flour for their noodles, as well as organic cheese. The brand I buy also happens to taste really good, so once in a while I eat some, too! And yes, it is a highly refined food, but until I have my very own vegan chef in the house, I will let the occasional indulgence pass by and trust that my kids will be back to eating fresh blueberries and snap peas before the day is over!

Chapter 24 - Xanthan Gum, et. al.

While I do admit the number of topics available for the letter X are few, there are a few things about xanthan gum I will share with you that may be important, so it's a win-win situation and all is well. I'll start with what it is.

Xanthan gum is a food additive most often found in processed foods. (To note, xanthan gum is also used in other industries, but my purpose here is food related, so I will not be writing about these other areas.) Its purpose is to enhance either the appearance, texture, or stability of food items.

Xanthan gum is created by a fermenting process using any of the following as the initial source: corn, wheat, soy, or whey. Anyone having food allergies or sensitivities to any of these four sources needs to know the source to make sure they are not affected by the finished product. Either that, or they may wish to skip food items processed with xanthan gum altogether. That said, it appears that xanthan gum derived from wheat is a gluten-free product, just in case you were wondering.

A concern for me that affects all of us is the fact that according to the USDA, as of 2012, 88% of corn and 94% of soy grown in the United States is genetically modified. The jury is out on whether or not genetically modified organisms (GMOs) are safe for human consumption. And there is currently no labeling requirement here in the U.S. for GMO products.

Add to that the fact that some of the conventional wheat crops grown in the U.S. are sprayed with a pervasive herbicide called glyphosate just before harvest. This routine allows for easier harvest of the wheat, but it also leaves a toxic residue on the grains that are used to make things like xanthan gum. Once again, you won't know this by reading the label.
If you have time to do the detective work, you will be able to find out the source of the xanthan gum in the products you may currently be eating. You may be able to find out if they are sourced from GMOs. It's not likely you'll learn whether chemical herbicides were used or not. If you don't wish to invest your time in said detective work, either choose an organic source, which cannot be GMO nor sprayed with glyphosate, or simply replace the questionable product with one that doesn't contain food additives. As with anything, organic is preferred. Otherwise, keep your eyes open for a "Non-GMO Project Verified"[11] rectangular blue seal on the label or packaging.

I'm going to use this space to make a point: Processed food items are full of additives that have questionable sources. Curious to know how many additives may be derived from corn? Check out this list:

1. Alpha tocopherol
2. Ascorbic acid
3. Baking powder
4. Calcium stearate
5. Caramel
6. Cellulose
7. Citric Acid
8. Citrus cloud emulsion

9. Corn flour
10. Corn oil
11. Cornstarch
12. Corn syrup
13. Dextrin
14. Dextrose (glucose)
15. Diglycerides
16. Ethylene
17. Ethyl acetate
18. Ethyl lactate
19. Fibersol-2
20. Fructose
21. Fumaric acid
22. Gluten
23. Golden syrup
24. High fructose corn syrup
25. Inositol
26. Invert sugar
27. Malt
28. Maltodextrin
29. Margarine
30. Monoglycerides
31. Monosodium glutamate (MSG)
32. Polydextrose
33. Saccharin
34. Semolina
35. Sorbic Acid
36. Sorbitol
37. Starch
38. Sucrose
39. Treacle
40. Vanilla extract
41. White vinegar
42. Xanthan gum
43. Xylitol
44. Zein

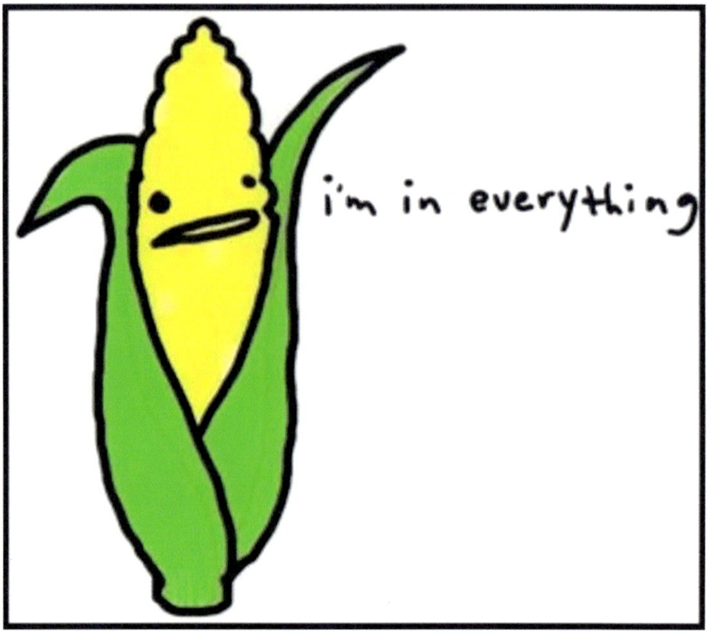

Would you believe this is the SHORT list? Anyway, I find it far easier to choose foods without these ingredients than to delve into the ingredient history of each product. By doing so, I know I am choosing better for myself and my family. I know you can succeed at this, too!

My best recommendation would be to choose one item in your pantry or refrigerator at a time and find a healthier replacement for it. Once you're comfortable with that change, replace another. After a few weeks, seeking out healthier products will become easier, and you will now be adding another block to the solid foundation of your and your family's future!

Chapter 25 - YOU!

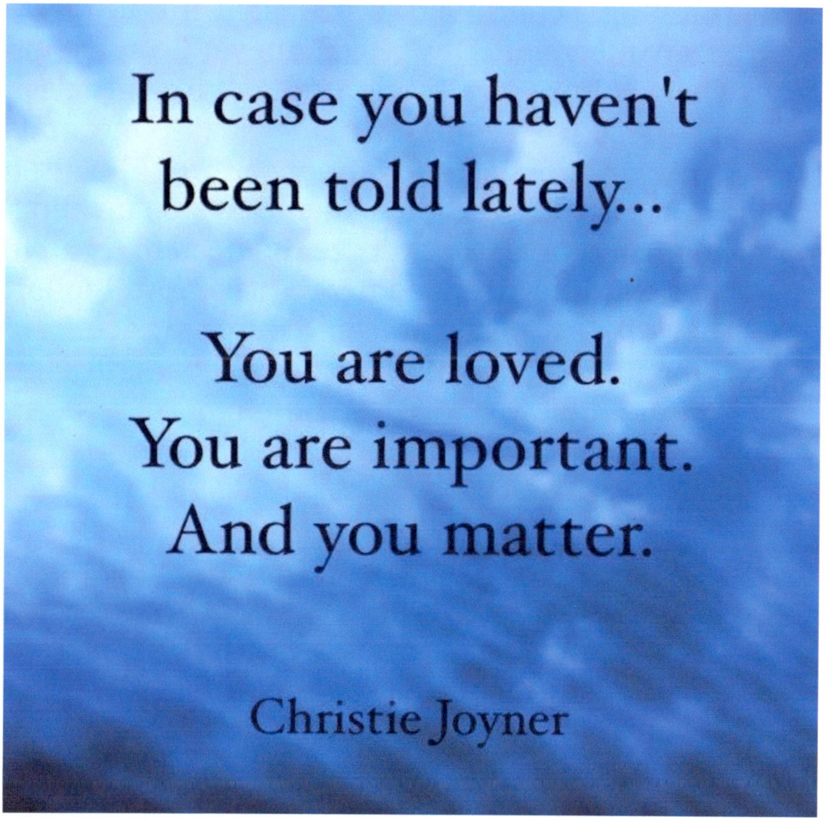

Perhaps you've heard it said - "a picture is worth a thousand words." In the case of the graphic above, it's quite possible these few words stir up in you what feels like a thousand emotions. It's also possible you don't believe them to be true. I know this, because there was a time in my life when my feelings of self-worth were "lower than whale poop," and I didn't feel as though anyone loved me, and no one could've convinced me I mattered at all. At the time, I was married with two small children. I had been verbally abused enough that I found myself questioning my core values and beliefs. Maybe I really was off the mark in my way of thinking. I continued to struggle with the disconnect in my marriage. Divorce had never been an option. There came a day, though, when my soul's desire to be free to live again was made clear to me, and I knew if I remained, my inner self would cease to exist. I asked my then husband to step up and seek help with me. He didn't see the need to fix anything, though, so he declined my request. And I followed that with my decision to end our marriage. Something inside of me had spoken loudly enough to remind me I was worth so much more!

And so are YOU!

YOU are so deserving of all that is good! Every idea you have is a wonderful product of your creativity! Every goal you have set is a worthy one! Every helping hand you offer is something to be proud of! And what to do if you haven't reached 100% confidence in your value and self-worth? I will share with you some things I have done to help me love myself and realize my own self-worth again. The truth is, if you don't love yourself, you cannot be completely available to love others as they deserve to be loved, including your children.
Interestingly enough, some of the techniques I used to heal myself began to trickle in to my life long before I would actually use them. This was in part due to my participation in educational events where I displayed the children's books I was selling as a vendor. I would meet other vendors, and learning

from them about energy healing techniques including reiki caused me to explore such topics on my own late into the evenings after my kids were in bed.

Aside from doing a lot of thinking, though, and not feeling any better, in my online searching I recall stumbling onto the website of a classical homeopathic doctor. He had two offices. One was in New York City, and as what I then considered to be luck would have it, his other office was in a town just two hours to the south of me. I was compelled to make an appointment with him, and that first three-hour appointment was the beginning of real change in my life. He helped me to unwrap what we decided to call my "shawl of oppression." In other words, he helped me begin to release my belief that my actions must meet the satisfaction of all those around me. Doing so was an impossible task, anyway, and it certainly had me giving myself little to no attention at all!

I recall having at least two follow up appointments with him. At the last of these, he asked me about my dreams for my life. After we talked for a bit, he offered me a ticket to attend an upcoming event in Chicago, IL, USA. He suggested that if I was thinking of attending, I should find a copy of The Secrets of the Millionaire Mind and read it first. So, I did. And then I worked out the details so I could attend The Millionaire Mind Intensive, a free three-day event 200 miles from my home and my children.

What I gained from attending was more than some excellent, easy-to-implement money managing skills. Until I attended this event I had no idea how "stuck" I was in beliefs I had learned as a child that were no longer serving me. There was one activity in which I released so much stuck energy that I cried and cried for several minutes. It seemed the start of a very embarrassing experience, but the people around me only supported me with hugs, kind words, and tissues. I have come to welcome these moments of release when they occur, and yes, they do still occur. I cannot predict when they are going to happen, but I always feel so much more free, as if weights I've been unknowingly carrying have been lifted away, after they pass.

As I continued my journey, I was given the opportunity to have a reiki session with someone I consider a friend. This session turned into more of a balancing session. To this day, I am no expert in balancing, which works with the energies of the seven chakras found within the human body. And while I did have a useful experience, it was the book she lent to me that I am offering here: Life! Reflections on Your Journey by Louise L. Hay. Louise offered compassionate words that helped me learn to honor my inner self and befriend the little girl who lives inside of me. And whether that sounds odd to you or not, know this: EVERYTHING will begin to shift to a better space when you learn to love yourself first!

While I was learning new things, I still stumbled, many times. I wasn't used to asking for help, and I often carried my burdens in silence. I don't recommend this. It is far better to build a village of caring people who will help you on your journey. If you don't find the support you need in person, you will absolutely be able to find it online. There are many motivational groups on Facebook, and if you keep the positive posts flowing through your newsfeed, the words you may need to hear the most will be there when you need them!

I found one such group when I began to explore meditation. I signed up for a 21-day meditation experience offered by the Chopra Center. I highly recommend meditation, and if you're new to the process, this experience will help you build a solid foundation. Meditation - Find the Quiet (if you haven't read that one yet!) goes into more detail about meditation when you're ready.

There was yet another supposed coincidence when I came across an email in my inbox asking me if I would be interested in speeding up the reprogramming of my subconscious mind so I might begin to enjoy new levels of success. I was absolutely interested in that! I talked with my kids and let them know how important it was for me to learn what this webinar had to teach. They were okay with going to bed a bit earlier than usual. I sat and watched the webinar. I knew without question I wanted to invest in myself and purchase the program that was being offered. That was in early 2011. I still have access to Winning the Game of Money, a program created by John Assaraf. And while I haven't topped the scales as a billionaire just yet, I have made sound advances in my financial life as well as my life in general. Within a year of having purchased this program, John offered another series of two programs regarding fear and procrastination. I bought these as well, and I promptly procrastinated and didn't use either of them for another three years! Personally, I recommend Winning the Game of Fear before any other program. It is one of my top three systems when it comes to making positive changes. It has made a significant difference in my life!

I have to make a connection here between John Assaraf, his appearance in a book/movie titled The Secret, and the law of attraction. Those happenings

I've referenced along the way as luck or coincidence, well, I no longer believe that's what they were. I believe that as you focus on your journey, those things, people, or ideas necessary for your advancement will appear for you as you are ready for them. It is not necessary to hold this belief. I am simply letting you know this is my belief.
My most recent gains have come from two additional areas of interest. The first of these is the emotional freedom technique (EFT), also known as tapping. I have dedicated chapter 5 to EFT, a very simple, effective, free tool for clearing energy blocks.
The second is not a technique but rather a person. Brendon Burchard is an incredible individual who has dedicated his life to motivating others to achieve their greatest potential through high performance actions and intentional living. His work is available in his books as well as through his online programs. I recently attended his High Performance Academy Live! event, and I will always refer to it as life-altering. Figurative ceilings were shattered at this event, and the energy levels were so high it only takes a moment, a song, or a memory to recapture that energy and remind myself that I am ready to achieve my dreams. I know it is truly my time to not only reach for the stars, but to touch them!
I know what has worked to build my inner strength and set me on the path to my highest potential may or may not resonate with you. I only hope to shorten your learning curve - if something I've mentioned does strike an inclination inside of you, give it a try. Just like the rest of this book, take what works and use it! If it holds no appeal for you, leave it behind. Only you know what the best options for you might be!

Chapter 26 - Zucchini ... and Other Suspect Fruits and Veggies

"Ever wonder why food is being made and modified by the world's largest pesticide manufacturer?" ~ GMO-Awareness

As I've been writing this book, I've mentioned genetically modified organisms (GMOs) here and there. This chapter is dedicated to presenting current information on GMOs. As time passes, I am sure this information will need updating. My hope is that the updates will be in favor of our health and not otherwise.

Aside from the fact they are present at all, the greatest difficulty with GMOs in the United States stems from the fact that the resulting products do not require a label telling consumers these products contain GMO ingredients. I believe we deserve the right to make informed choices about the foods we feed our families. Unfortunately, the U.S. lags behind more than 60 other countries which have made GMO labeling mandatory. JustLabelIt.org depicts the imbalance in this image, showing those countries that do not require labeling in blue:

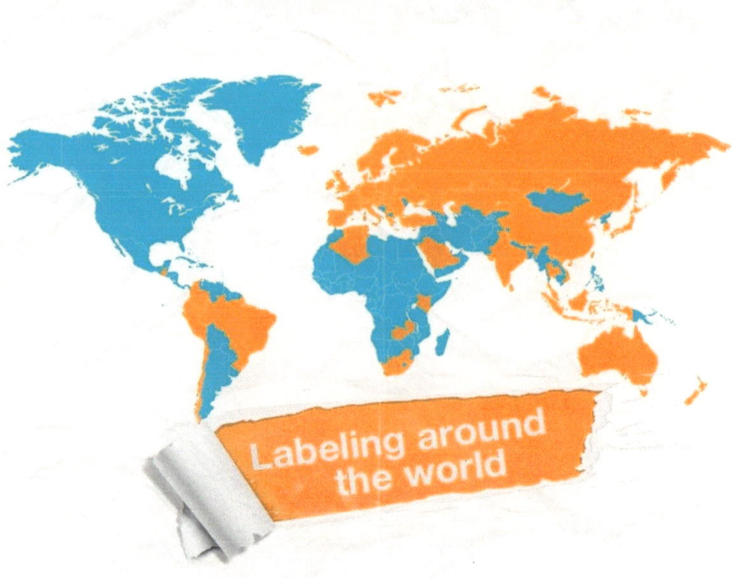

Currently, these crops, followed by their corresponding USDA-published percentages, are GMO here in the United States:

1. Corn - 92%
2. Cotton - 93%
3. Soybean - 94%
4. Sugar Beets - 90%
5. Canola - 88%
6. Hawaiian Papaya - 50%
7. Zucchini - unknown
8. Alfalfa - unknown

Food for thought:

- There is a list of ingredients in Chapter 24 that are potentially made from corn. There is a 92% chance these ingredients are GMO if they're not organic.
- How many of your clothes are made from cotton?
- It could be that one of your favorite bags of potato chips is made with cottonseed oil.
- Check out Chapter 15 for healthier oil options. Skip the canola!
- Soy protein is widely used in processed foods.
- If the sugar you purchase doesn't say it's cane sugar, it likely contains sugar made from sugar beets.
- You may not eat alfalfa, but many cows do. And you might eat beef or dairy products that come from these cows.

Genetic modification takes place when a specific gene from one species is forcibly inserted into a completely unrelated species. This is different than hybridization, which takes place between related species and has been occurring without ill effect for centuries. Interestingly enough, the primary reasons given for the genetic modification of food - increased yields, enhanced drought resistance, and improved nutrition - haven't become reality at all.
What has happened is one of two things: Crops have either been genetically modified to produce their own internal pesticides to either kill or deter insects, or they have been modified to withstand the herbicides that the SAME companies who are responsible for the genetic modifications happen to manufacture. These herbicides include glyphosate

(Roundup), glufosinate, and 2-4,D (an ingredient in Agent Orange).

While I do realize we are not insects, both insects and we ARE living creatures, and if the pesticides inherent to GMO sweet corn are designed to cause the belly of a corn earworm to explode, I'm not interested in eating the same corn and finding out whether my belly will be affected or not. The effects are more likely to be chronic than acute, meaning they will not show up immediately after eating said corn, but somewhere down the road as things build up in our systems. Truthfully, GMOs only have a twenty-year history, and there hasn't been any research done using humans as test subjects. I have no desire to be a human guinea pig. How about you?

Getting back to the second of these two genetic modifications, "Roundup Ready" crops, shows the implications to our health here are even worse. Glyphosate has recently been indicted as one of the most harmful chronic toxins in our environment and may indeed be the most important factor in the development of many chronic diseases and conditions. Dr. Rosemary Mason[12] says this about glyphosate's toxicity to human health:

"Glyphosate is an endocrine-disruptor, as are many herbicides. It damages DNA and it is a driver of mutations that lead to cancer. We present graphs from the US which correlate glyphosate application and the percentage of GE corn and soy crops to the incidence and prevalence of various diseases in those on a Western diet."

"The Pearson's correlation coefficients are very strong and highly significant for obesity, diabetes, autism, thyroid cancer, liver cancer, death from Parkinson's, Senile Dementia and Alzheimer's, inflammatory bowel disease and acute kidney

failure. We present Cancer Research UK graphs of upward trends in cancer incidences between 1975 and 2009, which are in line with the US graphs. Other consequences are gastrointestinal disorders, heart disease, depression, infertility, birth defects and other cancers."

Knowing these things, here is another tidbit to consider: When GM alfalfa was approved in late 2011, 93% of the alfalfa crops were not using ANY herbicide at all. There was no need to engineer an herbicide-resistant crop of alfalfa. It was predicted GM alfalfa would contaminate previously non-GMO crops. It did. And this leads to a whole host of other problems caused by genetically modified organisms. The dark hole of GMOs is a deep one.

My intent is to make sure you know they're out there. The question is, are you willing to change your habits and make healthier choices? Here are a few ideas to help you if you are, some of which I've mentioned earlier in this book:

1. Choose whole foods. Make sure they're organic if they're on the list of GMO crops. (Chapter 23)
2. Cook from scratch, again choosing ingredients you know to be non-GMO. Schedule a block of time to prepare meals for the week. Freeze accordingly.
3. Choose certified organic foods.
4. Choose foods bearing the "Non-GMO Project Verified"[13] label.
5. Use Internet resources to help make the transition easier:
    - http://www.nongmoshoppingguide.com/download.html
    - http://www.nongmoproject.org

6. Grow your own food. (Chapter 7)
7. Resource local foods. Meet your farmers. Talk with them to be sure they are growing to meet your standards! (Chapter 11)

The subject of genetically modified foods is a weighty one. There is a lot to consider, and it takes time to sort through all of the information available. Please hang in there! Eating well is very possible!
I also understand it can be challenging to find an awesome variety of high quality foods depending on your location and the time of the year. I live in a small town of less than 20,000 people in a northern climate, and only during July through October is the selection of high quality produce better than mundane. During these months it's worth taking some time to prepare and store extra fruits and veggies for the winter. If that seems like too great a challenge right now, other options include the following:

1. http://www.localharvest.org/
2. Join a wholesale buying club. Reach out to them and ask if there is a food buying club in your area. They will be able to give you an answer. Every food club has its own rules. What you will receive in return for your participation is an excellent selection of foods at wholesale prices. Here are two that I am aware of:
    - https://www.azurestandard.com/ (has fresh produce)
    - https://www.unfi.com/Pages/default.aspx (no fresh produce)

I am going to close the subject of GMOs by offering a resource entitled "GMO Myths and Truths: An evidence-based examination of the claims made for the safety and efficacy of genetically modified crops." It is a well-referenced resource that offers you more in-depth information if that is what you are seeking. Go here to see it: http://earthopensource.org/wordpress/downloads/GMO-Myths-and-Truths-edition2.pdf

About Me

Debbie Hagedorn currently works as a grower on a 400-acre farm in Wisconsin while she perseveres to create the business her entrepreneurial spirit has desired for many years. After the birth of her first child in 2002, Debbie found herself researching options that would provide a truly safe and healthy home for her family. She continues to add pertinent information into what she refers to as "the file box in my brain" on a regular basis. She uses this information to create products that assist others in making healthier choices in their lives without having to do all of the research first. 26 Ideas For Positive Change is her first book. You will find value and opportunities for further learning at her website: www.LiveWithVigor.com. She also welcomes you to visit her on Facebook at her page: Live With Vigor.

Endnotes

[1] http://www.livestrong.com/article/370945-health-effects-of-yellow-5-food-coloring/

[2] http://articles.mercola.com/sites/articles/archive/2010/03/02/old-monsanto-food-toxin-disguised-under-new-name.aspx

[3] http://www.livestrong.com/article/288335-the-most-common-food-preservatives/

[4] http://foodmatters.tv/articles-1/top-10-food-additives-to-avoid

[5] http://www.nytimes.com/2012/07/18/science/fda-bans-bpa-from-baby-bottles-and-sippy-cups.html

[6] http://fluoridealert.org/issues/water/fluoridation-chemicals/

[7] http://articles.mercola.com/sites/articles/archive/2013/12/21/9-farmed-fish-facts.aspx

[8] http://www.choosemyplate.gov/index.html

[9] http://www.choosemyplate.gov/printpages/MyPlateFoodGroups/ProteinFoods/food-groups.protein foods-amount.pdf

[10] http://articles.mercola.com/sites/articles/archive/2013/12/22/dr-holick-vitamin-d-benefits.aspx

[11] http://www.nongmoproject.org/

[12] http://www.gmoevidence.com/dr-mason-glyphosate-is-destructor-of-human-health-and-biodiversity/

[13] http://www.nongmoproject.org

Made in the USA
Monee, IL
05 November 2026

67384874R00071